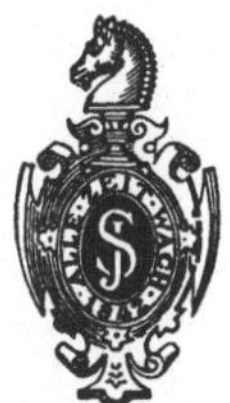

Recent Results in Cancer Research

Fortschritte der Krebsforschung

Progrès dans les recherches sur le cancer

30

Edited by

Editor in chief

P. Rentchnick, Genève

1970

Springer-Verlag Berlin Heidelberg GmbH 1970

Advances in the Treatment of Acute (Blastic) Leukemias

Edited by

Georges Mathé

With 84 Figures

1970

Springer-Verlag Berlin Heidelberg GmbH 1970

Proceedings of the plenary session of the European Organization for Research on Treatment of Cancer (E.O.R.T.C.) and its cooperative groups. Paris, June 1969

Georges Mathé, Professor de Cancérologie Expérimentale à la Faculté de Médecine de Paris. Directeur de l'Institut de Cancérologie et d'Immunogénétique, Hôpital Paul-Brousse, F-94 Villejuif

Sponsored by the Swiss League against Cancer

ISBN 978-3-662-34998-4
DOI 10.1007/978-3-662-35334-9
ISBN 978-3-662-35334-9 (eBook)

Title No. 3645

Preface

The 1969 Proceedings of the Plenary Session of the European Organization for Research on Treatment of Cancer have been divided between two volumes of a completely different nature.

Volume 29, Aseptic Environments and Cancer Treatment, deals not only with the treatment of all types of cancer but also with aplastic treatment of bone marrow and certain other pathological conditions, such as immunological insufficiency, burns etc. Hence the volume will be of interest not only to carcinologists and haematologists but also to paediatricians, surgical units, intensive-care units, hospital administrators and architects and engineers who specialize in hospital design and equipment.

Volume 30, Advances in the Treatment of Acute (Blastic) Leukemias, deals with a particular form of cancer and will have a more restricted readership of carcinologists specializing in leukemia and all haematologists.

Paris, April 1970 GEORGES MATHÉ

Contents

I. Means and Methods

A. Daunomycin

B. Asparaginase

C. Dioxopiperazine Propane

D. Other Drugs

E. Immunotherapy

II. Strategy of the Treatment

III. Blastic Leukemias Secondary to Chronic Leukemias and Lymphomas

IV. Conclusions

Introduction

D. W. van Bekkum

President of the EORTC

The European Organization for Research on Treatment of Cancer (EORTC) has only a short history.

Nearly 7 years ago a small group of people, among them laboratory researchers as well as clinical oncologists from a number of European countries, came together and decided to start an effort towards European collaboration in the broad field of cancer treatment.

During the first few years the group's activities concentrated on the screening of chemical compounds for tumor-inhibiting properties and on the organization of clinical cooperative groups for the evaluation of new drugs in the treatment of various forms of cancer in patients.

Soon the group's adopted name, Groupe Européen de Chimiothérapie Anticancéreuse (GECA), became a widely recognized trademark, which had to be changed to EORTC in 1968, when it became clear that the potentialities of cooperation between the members and within the cooperative groups went beyond the limited field of cancer chemotherapy. Supportive cooperative groups engaged in more fundamental aspects of cancer research have been started and the members of the group have recognized the advantages of combining their efforts in other fields of research on the treatment of cancer, such as immunotherapy, radiotherapy and experimental oncology.

The present range of activities of EORTC and its associated cooperative groups can be summarized as follows.

1. Screening of substances for their anti-cancer activity using in vitro and in vivo screens. Secondary testing of specific compounds for other biological properties, such as immune suppression. More than 650 compounds have been processed so far.

2. Collaboration between clinical centers engaged in the treatment of cancer by way of the organization of clinical cooperative groups on a variety of forms of cancer. So far 10 clinical cooperative groups have been established and many of them have already produced important reports.

3. Organization of collaborative research between a number of research laboratories and departments of clinical medicine throughout Europe.

It should be mentioned here that the publication of the European Journal of Cancer, starting in 1965, has been an initiative of the EORTC and much of what is being achieved in the way of scientific research by EORTC associated workers can be found on the pages of that journal.

In looking back over the EORTC's achievements many inadequacies are still apparent, but it seems to me that we have succeeded in at least one direction, namely in abolishing various borders and barriers that have stood in the way of cancer research in Europe. I am not only referring to borders between the various nations, but also to barriers that separated the clinicians and the scientists and even different groups in one and the same country.

One tradition of the EORTC is that it attempts to organize once a year a meeting for all cancerologists at which its members and its cooperative groups present their results. This year is an important one for our organization. Not only will the meeting extend over two full days, but its program marks a serious attempt to abolish yet another barrier: that between the United States and Europe. Transatlantic cooperation will clearly be the next step in the collaborative investigation of cancer treatment.

Today, speakers from the leading centers in the United States as well as from Europe will compare and integrate their results and their visions, and, which is even more interesting, critically evaluate each other's conclusions.

It is my honour to express our thanks to Monsieur Galley, Minister of Scientific Research of France, for his kindness to sponsor our meeting.

We gratefully acknowledge the support of the CNRS in providing the present excellent meeting facilities and last but not least I wish to congratulate my friend Georges Mathé for his admirable achievement in the organization of the program and the many other activities that go with it. EORTC is lucky to have him, as one of the initiators of the group and its past president, continue to give us his unlimited interest and support.

I welcome all the participants and look forward to a fruitful and stimulating conference.

I. Means and Methods

A. Daunomycin

Present Results on Daunorubicine

(Rubidomycin, Daunomycin)

JEAN BERNARD, C. JACQUILLAT, M. WEIL, M. BOIRON, and J. TANZER

Institut de Recherches sur les Leucémies, Hôpital Saint-Louis, Paris

With 1 Figure

We have treated 1299 patients with Daunorubicine between 1966 and 1969 (Table 1). Among those patients 785 were treated at the Hôpital Saint Louis with our personal protocols, 514 were treated according to protocols of ALGB. I am glad to have this opportinuty to thank Dr. J. F. HOLLAND for his chairmanship and for his friendship.

We would like in this presentation to recall already well known facts (activity of Daunorubicine on advanced acute lymphoblastic leukemias resistant to other drugs, induction of complete remissions in A. M. L. at a higher rate than with other drugs), we will also report results of more recent studies dealing with combinations of Daunorubicine with other drugs.

Two facts are well established. The risk of typical cardiac accidents with high doses (above 30 mg/kg within 5 months) (Table 2) and the relative rarity of such accidents at lower doses (Table 3).

However many questions remain unanswered. Is the cardiac risk as severe if total high doses are distributed within a long period of time 2 years, 3 years or more. This eventuality will be met in protocols including so called "reinduction".

Which is the responsability of Rubidomycine in the origin of equivocal accidents for which there may be other explanations (cardiac history—collapsus with sepsis). It should be outlined that these accidents are more frequent in elderly patients and are seen more often in males than in females.

That Daunorubicine may induce complete remissions in A. L. L. resistant to other drug has been confirmed since 1966 by many publications.

But the most striking feature of Daunorubicin is the ability to induce a relativity high rate of C. R. in A. M. L. as it has been already shown at the international symposium on Rubidomycin in Paris in 1967.

Table 1. *Number of patients treated by rubidomycine alone or combinated to other drugs*

Rubidomycine alone	AML	Phase 1	64			
	ALL	relapses	38			
	6706	ALGB		(27)	129	
	6706 A	ALGB		(36)	211	
	6806	ALGB		(12)	65	
	LMC	Phase 1	16			
	Hodgkin	Phase 1	6			
Combinations	06 LA 66		130			
	6801	ALGB		(33)	109	
	06 LA 66 01 LA 67 02 LA 67 02 LA 68	relapses of ALL	270			
	06 LA 66 LBS		50			
	Quintuple		50			
	RU+MTX		17			
	RU+Aase		9			
	Epitheliomas		135			
	Total		785	(108)	514	1299

June 1969.

Table 2. *Deaths from cardio toxicity. Observed in A. L. treated with rubidomycin*

Leukemia	Total dose (mg/kg)	Interval between beginning of treatment and first cardiac troubles
LAL, 6 y.	42	5 months
LAM, 10 y.	40	6 months
LAL, 6 y.	32	5 months
LAL, 10 y.	42	5 months
LAL, 8 y.	45	6 months

Table 3. *Cardiac toxicity*

	Number of patients	Unequivocal cardiac toxicity	Equivocal cardiac toxicity
> 30 mg/kg	13	5	
< 30 mg/kg	1010	2	22
Total	1023	7	22

Table 4. *Protocol Paris 06 LA 66*

Pred. 100 $mg/m^2/d.$ Vinc. 2 $mg/m^2/w.$ Rub. 60 $mg/m^2/w.$	→ RC → Maintenance { 6MP 90 $mg/m^2/d.$; Mtx 15 $mg/m^2/w.$ } +Mtx IT/m 10 mg/m^2
	+Reinductions { Pred. 100 $mg/m^2 \times 7$ d.; Vinc. 2 $mg/m^2/d.$ 1 and 7; Rub. 30 $mg/m^2/d.$ 1 and 7; Mtx IT—2 Inj. 10 mg/m^2 } ↓ At 0.5, 1, 2, 4, 7, 11, 16 months → ev. 6 months

Table 5. *Results obtained with daunorubicin in induction. Treatment for acute myelocytic leukaemia*

Result	1st attack		1st relapse		2nd relapse		3rd relapse		Total
	Children	Adults	Children	Adults	Children	Adults	Children	Adults	
Complete remission	6	20	3	3	1	1	1	0	35
Partial remission	0	4	1	1	0	1	1	0	8
No improvement	1	12	0	5	2	1	0	0	21
Total	7	36	4	9	3	3	2	0	64

In our experience, the maximum daily dose was 2 mg/kg; the number of doses and duration of treatment varied from one case to another depending on the decrease of white blood cells and the modifications of bone marrow smears, the percentage of blast cells and cellularity being especially taken in consideration. On the whole the mean number of doses was 7 and the mean total dose given was 12 mg/kg.

In the first 64 patients with acute granulocytic leukemias treated according to the protocol indicated on Table 4, 35 complete remissions were attained (Table 5); more remissions were obtained in children than in adults. All patients suffered a severe aplasia and most of the patients who did not attain remission died during induction phase from bleeding or still more frequently from sepsis. These aplasias are the main draw back of Daunorubicine.

In these 35 patients the median remission time has been 155 days; in four cases however it lasted more than two years and 2 of these patients are still in remission after two and half years: both were promyelocytic forms and we must emphasize the striking sensitivity to Daunorubicine of these forms formerly the most severe of all.

We shall now consider combinations with Rubidomycine: in A. L. L. Rubidomycine has been added since 1967 to the program that we apply at the Hôpital Saint Louis since 1963. This program combines an induction treatment with Vincristine and Prednisone, a maintenance treatment with continuous 6-MP and intermittent Methotrexate, and systematic "reinduction" courses at definite intervals.

Table 6. *Treatment of AML with rubidomycin Paris protocol*

Induction	Maintenance	Reinductions
Ru. 60 mg/m² 2—7 days	6-MP 90 mg/m²/d. Mtx 15 mg/m²/w.	1, 2, 4, 7, 11 months Ru. 30 mg/m²/days 1 and 8 M. GAG. 350 mg/m²/days 3 and 5

Table 7. *Protocole 06 LA 66 (Paris). Mars 1967, coloque international sur la rubidomycine*

	Enfants	Adultes	Total
R. C.	17	8	25
R. I.			
Echecs		3	3
Total	17	11	28

Table 8. *Results of combination of L-asparaginase. Vincristine rubidomycine prednisone in ALL*

Number of cases	1st attack	1st relapse	2nd relapse	3rd relapse	4th or 5th relapse	Total
Complete remissions		13 (6)	4 (3)	2	2 (1)	21 (10)
Partial remissions			1			1
Partial failure		1				1
Total failure		1 (1)				1 (1)
Death on treatment		3 (2)				3 (2)
Total		18 (9)	5 (3)	2	2 (1)	27 (13)

Between brackets figure the patients with prior treatment of Prednisone—Vincristine—Rubidomycine. June 1969.

The interest of these inducer doses is proved by our results and also by those of two independant protocols of ALGB; ALGB 6413 and ALGB 6601.

It is not our intention to detail these results but 25% of the patients treated according to he protocol initiated in 1964 are still in remission between the forth and the fifth year. Those datas are impressive if one considers that until now the frequency of remissions lasting more than 5 years was evaluated approximately at 1%.

Protocol Paris 6606 is indicated on Table 6.

The first results, presented at the "International Symposium on Rubidomycin" in March 1967 showed a high rate of remissions. Complete remissions are obtained with high frequency in adults, in very young people (less than 1 year) and in forms with high leucocytosis. In one patient who attained complete remission, white blood cells count was 1 600 000 (Table 7).

Fig. 1 shows the initial comparison of protocols 02 LA 64 and 04 LA 65 (which differ only by the frequency of induction doses) and protocol 6606.

Studies on the combination of Vincristine, Daunorubicine, Asparaginase and Prednisone are pursued on relapses as well as on first attacks and complete remissions are

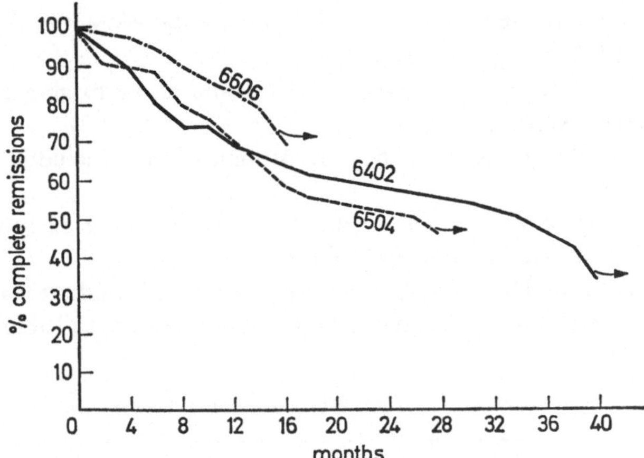

Fig. 1. Duration of first complete remission in children ≦ 15 years. — 6402 (41 c.), - - - 6504 (38 c.); —·—·— 6606 (87 c.)

Table 9. *Acute granulocytic leukemias*

Induction treatment	Years	No. of cases	No. of C. R.	% of C. R.
Pr+MTX	1956—1960	118	17	14
6-MP+GAG	1963	45	14	33
6-MP+GAG+MTX	1964	24	9	35
Ara-C	1965	39	12	30
Ara-C+GAG+6-MP+Pr	1966	37	13	35
Total	1956—1966	263	65	23

> 4 years, 7 cases. June 1969.

Table 10. *Acute granulocytic leukemias*

Rubidomycine		Years	No. of cases	No. of C. R.	% of C. R.
		1967	64	35	54
ALGB	A (3 days)		45	13	29
6706	B (5 days)	1968	49	11	22
	C (7 days)		31	7	22
ALGB	A (5 days)		61	21	34
6706 A	B (b; w.)	1968	62	13	21
	C (o. w.)		75	12	16
Ara-C+GAG+ 6-MP+RU+Pr		1968	32	13	40
6-MP+GAG +RU+Pr		1968	18	6	35
RU+MTX		1969	17	6	35
RU+MTX+Aase		1969	9	5	55
Total		1967—1969	463	142	32

June 1969

obtained with high frequency even in patient previously treated by the drugs already mentioned except l-Asparaginase (Table 8).

In A. M. L. the need of combination which would allow to give Daunorubicin at the less toxic doses is still more urgent.

Table shows results of various combinations some of them including Daunorubicine (Table 9 and Table 10).

Each of these combinations was tried with only one dose of each drug so that definite conclusion or desillusion would be erroneous.

The combination of Daunorubicine, Asparaginase and Methotrexate appeared to have some interest but it has to be confirmed by additional cases (Table 11).

Table 11. *Results of combination of L-asparaginase—rubidomycine—methotrexate in A. M. L.*

Number of cases	1st attack	1st relapse	2nd relapse	Total
C. R.	4+1 [a]	1		5+1 [a]
Partial remission				
Partial failure			1	1
Total failure	1			1
Total				8

[a] Death in C. R. on day 30. June 1969.

One may thus conclude that Rubidomycine is a significant aquisition in the treatment of acute leukemias. Its major toxic threat is marrow aplasia rather than cardiac toxicity which is important only at high doses, in elderly patients or in those who have a cardiac history.

Its future lies mainly in active combinations.

Summary

The present status of daunorubicin results is summarized.

This drug, given alone, induces a relatively high rate of complete remissions in A. M. L.

Cardiac toxicity does not seem to offer an excessive threat if daunorubicin administration is avoided in patients with a cardiac history and in elderly patients, and if total doses are below 30 mg/kg.

The major drawback of daunorubicin is the risk of severe irreversible aplasias.

Given in combination with vincristine and prednisone, daunorubicin induces a high rate of complete remissions in A. L. L. even in poor-risk patients.

Studies of combinations, of daunorubicin, vincristine, prednisone and L-asparaginase in A. L. L. are in progress.

In A. M. L. combinations of daunorubicin with the other active drugs (ara-C, méthyl-GAG, etc.) were tried.

A study of the combination of L-asparaginase and daunorubicin is in progress.

Rubidomycin (or Daunomycin): A Clinicial Evaluation

"Leukemia and Hematosarcoma" Cooperative Group [1] of the European Organisation for Research on the Treatment of Cancer (E.O.R.T.C.)

Secretaryship: Institut de Cancérologie et d'Immunogénétique, Hôpital Paul-Brousse 14, avenue Paul-Vaillant Couturier, 94-Villejuif

With 3 Figures

Since Rubidomycin or Daunomycin has been used in the treatment of acute leukemias its effectiveness and toxicity have been differently evaluated. It might be profitable to point out a few conclusions drawn from therapeutic trials carried out by the Leukemia Group of E.O.R.T.C. and by MATHÉ's group.

On Table 1, we can see that Daunomycin used alone is less effective than Prednisone or Vincristine.

Table 1. *Value of efficient drugs in acute lymphoblastic leukaemia to induce complete remissions*

Drugs	Frequency of complete remissions
Prednisone	58%
Vincristine	43%
Daunomycin	25%

[1] President: W. F. STENFERT-KROESE; Responsible for the E.O.R.T.C.: G. MATHÉ; Secretary: M. HAYAT. Members who have cooperated to this trial: ALLEMAGNE: S. WITTE, K. TH. SCHRICKER (Medizinische Klinik mit Poliklinik der Universität Erlangen-Nürnberg, Erlangen); BELGIQUE: H. TAGNON, Y. KENIS (Institut Jules Bordet, Bruxelles); P. BASTENIE, CH. CAUCHIE (Hôpital Saint-Pierre, Bruxelles); FRANCE: J. BOUSSER, G. BILSKI-PASQUIER, A. BERNADOU, C. M. BLANC, R. ZITTOUN (Hôpital de l'Hotel-Dieu, Paris); P. CROIZAT, L. REVOL, J. J. VIALA (Hôpital Edouard-Herriot, Lyon); G. MATHÉ, J. L. AMIEL, A. CATTAN, M. HAYAT. F. DE VASSAL, CL. JASMIN, CL. ROSENFELD, J. R. SCHLUMBERGER, M. SCHNEIDER, L. SCHWARZENBERG (Service d'Hématologie de l'Institut Gustave-Roussy et Institut de Cancérologie et d'Immunogénétique, 94-Villejuif; GRANDE-BRETAGNE: G. HAMILTON FAIRLEY, R. B. SCOTT, M. LIPSEDGE (Saint Bartholomew's Hospital, Londres); HOLLANDE: W. H. STENFERT-KROESE (Rotterdamsch Radiotherapeutisch Instituut, Rotterdam); IRLANDE: J. B. HEALY (Saint-Luke's Hospital, Dublin); ITALIE: R. BULGARELLI, L. MASSIMO (Istituto G. Caslini, Gênes); L. BUSSI, D. CIPRINANI (Ospedale Maggiore Ca'Grande, Milan); E. POLLI, G. SALA (Istituto de Semeiotica Medica, Milan).

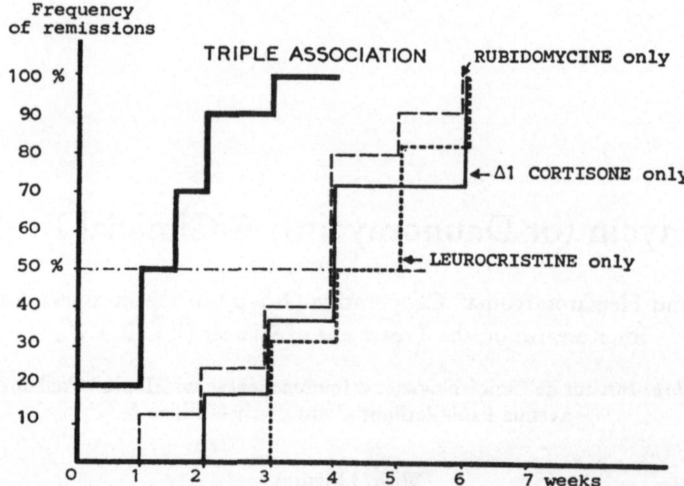

Fig. 1. Time taken by the association of Δ-1-cortisone, and rubidomycine, by leurocristine alone and Δ-1-cortisone alone to induce a complete remission

Table 2. *Effect of different schedules of treatment on acute lymphoblastic leukemia*

Drugs	Frequency of complete remission
Daunomycin	25%
Daunomycin +Vincristine +Prednisone	100% (children in primary acute leukemia) 85% (all cases)

Table 3. *Extremely severe aplasias during the first phase of complementary chemotherapy following remission*

Chemotherapy inducing remission	Number of patients	Number of aplasias
Prednisone +Vincristine	28	0
Prednisone +Vincristine +rubidomycin	59	11 (5 Deaths due to septicemia)

On the other hand (Table 2), in combination with Prednisone and Vincristine, we obtained an overall remission rate of 85%, and 100% in previously untreated children [4, 6].

Furthermore remissions were obtained much more rapidly than with either one of the drugs used alone. On the average, it takes 2 Weeks to achieve a remission (Fig. 1).

However, although this therapy is very effective, the aplasia resulting from Daunomycin is such that severe complications have occured shortly after beginning

Table 4. *Frequency of complete remission in acute myeloblastic leukaemia with daunomycin alone*

J. Bernard et al.	51%
G. Mathé et al.	25%
Children's cancer group A	0%
Leukaemia group of E.O.R.T.C	26%

Table 5. *Effect of daunomycin in acute granulocytic leukemias*

Detectable phase	Number of cases	Remissions		Failures	
		Complete	Incomplete	Not total	Total
1	43	13	7	6	17
2	27	5	4	5	13
3	1				1
Total	71	18	11	11	31

Table 6. *Effect of different schedules of treatment on acute granulocytic leukemia*

Drugs or associations	Frequency of complete remission
Daunomycin	25%
Daunomycin +Vincristine +Prednisone	26%
Daunomycin +Cytosine arabinoside +Prednisone +Methyl-GAG	25%

the consolidation therapy. 5 patients died of septicemia (Table 3) in spite of intensive supportive therapy including leucocyte transfusions. In view of this problem, we, no longer, use Daunomycin for induction chemotherapy.

As far as acute myeloblastic leukemia is concerned we can see that, with Daunomycin alone, different rates of complete remission have been reported (Table 4) [1, 2, 3].

On Table 5, we see the detail of E.O.R.T.C. trial where we obtained 26% complete remissions [5].

However in these myeloblastic leukemias as we can see (Table 6), the result is not improved by using Daunomycin in combination therapy.

Once again, we have to emphasize the toxicity of Daunomycin. We have already mentioned its marrow toxicity. The Table 7 shows that we had also 5 deaths due to acute cardiac failure. Its our impression that frequent electrocardiograms do not allow to foresee and avoid this complication.

On the other hand we found that determining the serum level of Creatinephosphokinase (C.P.K.) before each injection was useful in detecting early cardiac toxicity.

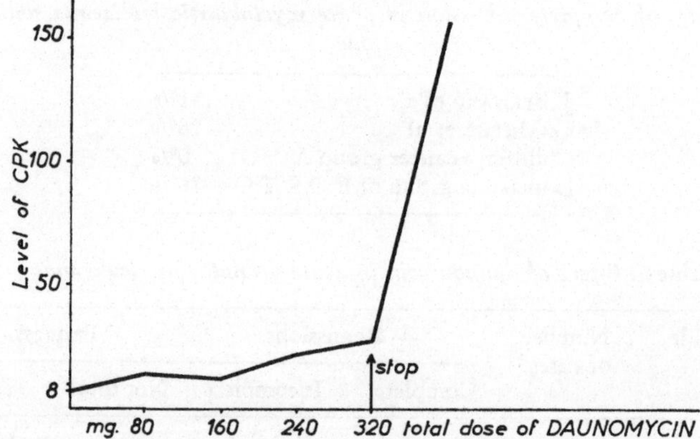

Fig. 2. Relation between the variation of CPK level and the dose of daunomycine in a patient with acute myeloblastic leukemia

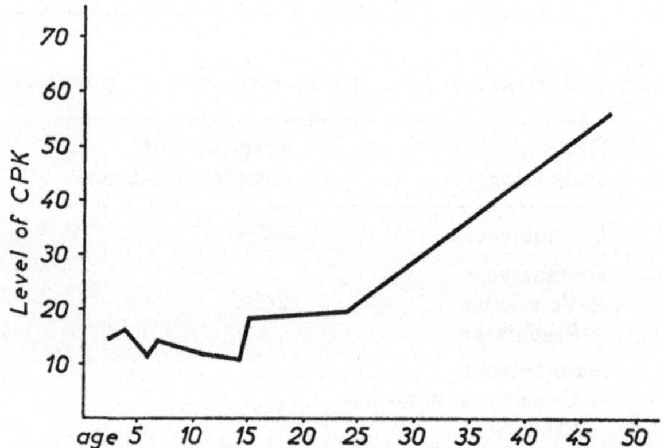

Fig. 3. Variation in function of age and of CPK level after a fixed dose of daunomycine (70 mg/m²)

Table 7. *Cardiovascular toxicity of daunomycin*

Number of cases studied	Minor manifestations	Major manifestations	Number of deaths
112	12	10	5

Table 8. *Variations in the level of creatine-phospho-kinase (CPK) during treatment with daunomycin*

Average level of CPK before treatment	Average level of CPK after an average total dose of 70 mg/m²	Statistic significance
10.6 U.	32.2 U.	$p < 0.05$

We recommend that Daunomycin be discontinued as soon as there is a significant increase in CPK level (Fig. 2). The Table 8 shows the median increase of CPK after a total dose of 70 mg/per square meter of Daunomycin. This rise in serum CPK Level, after the same total dose increase progressively with the age of patient (Fig. 3).

In summary, we feel that the usefulness of Daunomycin has been somewhat overestimated and is limited by its toxicity.

References

1. Boiron, M., Jaquillat, Cl., Weil, M., Thomas, M., Bernard, J.: Traitement des leucémies aiguës granulocytaires par la rubidomycine. Path. et Biol. **15**, 921 (1967).
2. Mathé, G., Hayat, M., Schwarzenberg, L., Schneider, M., Cattan, A., Schlumberger, J. R., Amiel, J. L.: Essai de traitement des leucémies aiguës par la rubidomycine (ou daunomycine) seule ou en association. Path. et Biol. **15**, 933 (1967).
3. Children's cancer group A — Preliminary evaluation of daunomycin in children with acute leukemia. Path. et Biol. **15**, 939 (1967).
4. Mathé, G., Hayat, M., Schwarzenberg, L., Amiel, J. L., Schneider, M., Cattan, A., Schlumberger, J. R., Jasmin, Cl.: Haute fréquence et qualité des rémissions de la leucémie aigue lymphoblastique chez l'enfant. Arch. franç. Pédiat. **25**, 181—188 (1968).
5. Organisation Européenne de Recherche sur le Traitement du Cancer — Groupe Coopérateur «Leucémies et Hématosarcomes» — Essai de traitement des leucémies aiguës granulocytaires par la daunomycine. J. Europ. Cancer **5**, 339 (1969).
6. Mathé, G., Schwarzenberg, L., Schneider, M., Schlumberger, J. R., Amiel, J. L., Cattan, A., Jasmin, Cl.: Acute lymphoblastic leukemia treated with a combination of prednisone, vincristine and rubidomycin. Lancet **2**, 380—383 (1967).

The Effect of Daunomycin on Proliferation and Survival of Human Leukemic Blasts in vivo

P. A. Strycкmans, J. Manaster, and M. Socquet

Department of Internal Medicine, Institut Jules Bordet, University of Brussels

With 5 Figures

Daunomycin or Rubidomycin is an antibiotic active against human acute leukemia [1]. It was shown to inhibit RNA and DNA synthesis [2, 3] and to produce an immediate reduction in the mitotic activity [4] in a variety of experimental tumors and mammalian cell lines.

The lethal effect of Daunomycin was found to be maximal during the DNA synthetic phase [5].

In order to find the best schedule of administration of Daunomycin, leukemic patients were investigated to determine where this drug is acting on the cell cycle on human leukemic blasts in vivo.

Methods

Six adults patients at the time of diagnosis of acute myeloblastic or monoblastic leukemia were given tritiated thymidine (^{3}HTdr) (0.1 μCi/g of body weight) (5 Ci/mMole) intravenously, 1 hour prior to administration of Daunomycin. A seventh patient with acute myeloblastic leukemia was given ^{3}HTdr 24 hours before Daunomycin. Daunomycin was given IV in a single injection of 70 or 80 mg/m^2. A first sample of bone marrow (BM) and blood were taken from all the patients 1 hour after ^{3}HTdr. Serial samples were drawn thereafter for several days. All the samples were processed for autoradiography (ARG). The labeling index of the leukemic blasts (LI) was determined by counting the number of labeled nuclei in at least 1,000 blasts.

For two patients, 200 BM blasts at 1, 24 and 48 hours were photographed and transparencies were projected on a screen. Two perpendicular diameters were measured for each projected blast nucleus.

Results

As a consequence of Daunomycin, the absolute number of blasts in the peripheral blood showed an immediate or somewhat delayed drop which was exponential for some time.

Percent of the number of circulating blasts before Daunomycin
T 1/2=11h
T 1/2=9 h
T 1/2=7h
T 1/2=8h
Hours after i.v. Daunomycin
Fig. 1

Percent of the initial labeling index in the blood
Daunomycin
Daunomycin
Hours after 3HTdr
Fig. 2

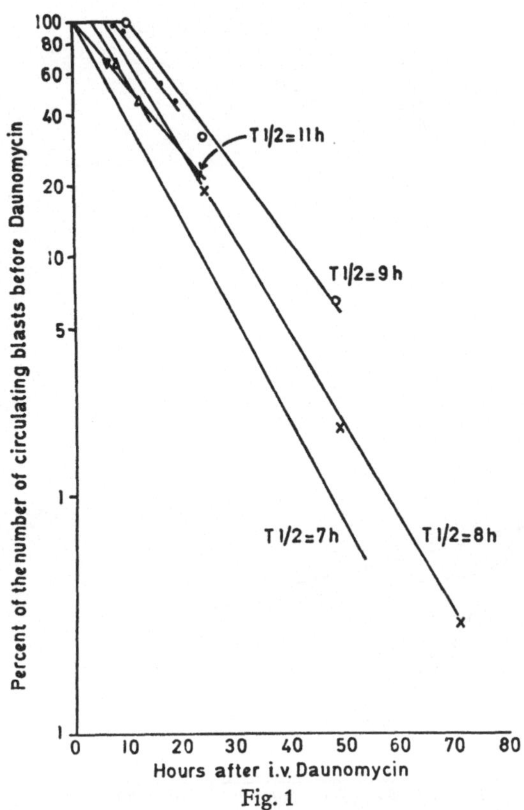

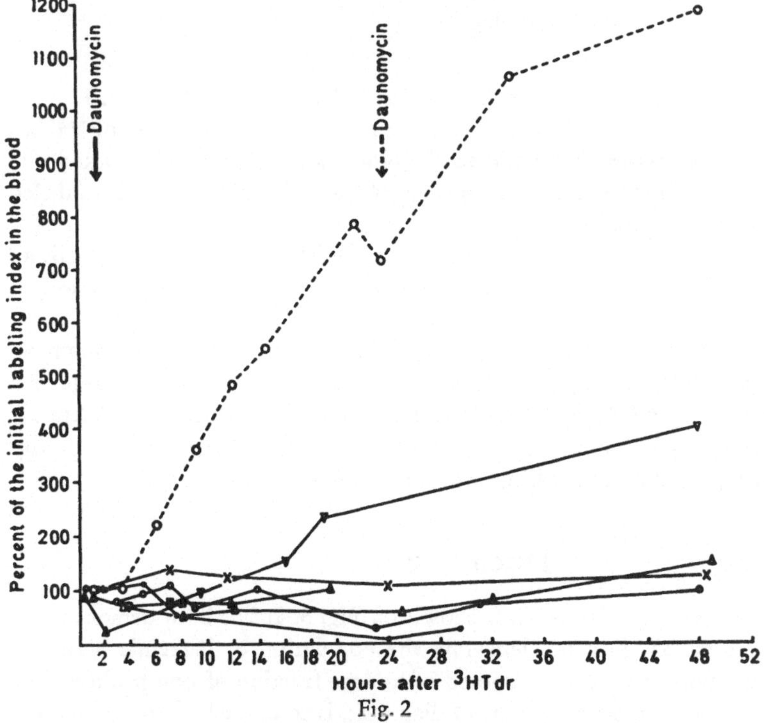

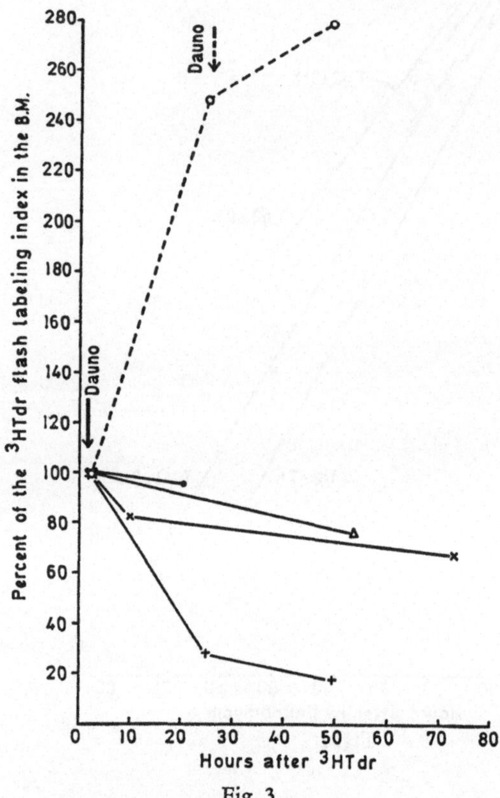

Fig. 3

The $T^1/_2$ was for all patients of the order of 8 to 11 hours as shown in Fig. 1.

Fig. 2 shows that when Daunomycin was given right after the injection of ^{3}HTdr, the release of labeled blasts from the BM to the blood was immediately blocked. On the other hand, when Daunomycin was injected 24 hours later than ^{3}HTdr, labeled BM blasts could still be released to the blood.

Fig. 3 shows that without Daunomycin the LI of the BM blasts increased. Such an increase was not seen when Daunomycin was given 1 hour after the injection of ^{3}HTdr.

The distribution of BM blasts according to the size of their nuclei is shown on Fig. 4. The labeled blasts are represented black and are confined to the large size categories. Twenty-four and 48 hours after Daunomycin, the labeled cells disappear progressively, but remain into the large size categories. Within 24 to 48 hours, initially unlabeled cells enlarge and enter the large size categories.

Discussion

A current model for acute leukemia is shown on Fig. 5. It has been demonstrated by many investigators that in acute leukemia the population of leukemic blasts, as other neoplastic cell populations, is composed of a large fraction of non proliferating cells. The BM blast population, at the time of diagnosis, is composed of approximately

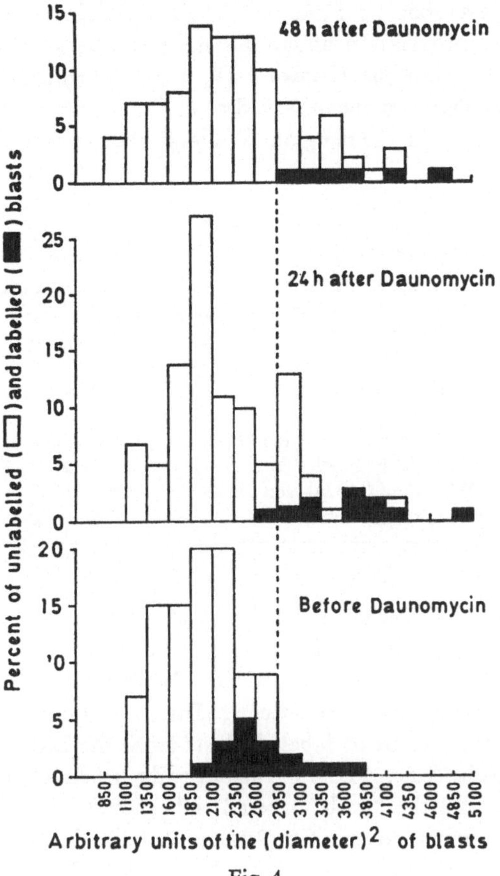

Fig. 4

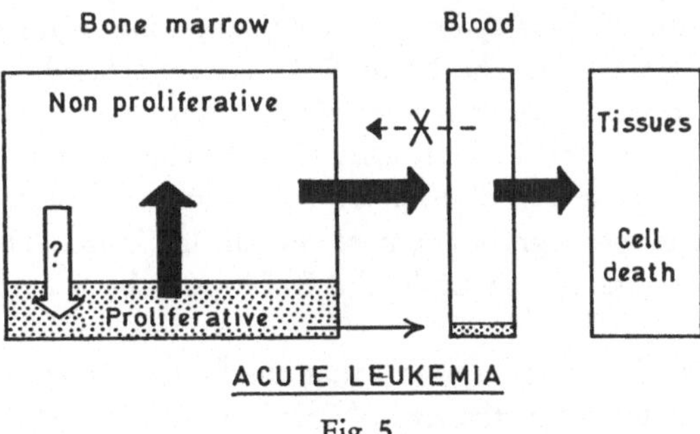

Fig. 5

$^1/_5$ of proliferating blasts and $^4/_5$ of non proliferating blasts. After one or successive divisions, the proliferating cells of the BM are preferentially released to the blood [7, 8]. Blood blasts are almost exclusively non proliferating [8].

If one hypothesize that the only effect of Daunomycin would be to block the release of leukemic blasts from the BM to the blood, then the $T^1/_2$ of leukemic blasts in the blood should be as short as the natural T½ of blood blasts in untreated leukemia. There is only scarce information about this natural T½ as shown on Table 1. All available information from the literature [9, 10, 11], whatever the method used, indicate a T½ longer than the one observed after Daunomycin. This can be explained only by a cytocidal effect of the drug on the blood blast cells which are mainly of the non-proliferating variety.

Table 1. *Half time of blood leukemic blasts*

	Untreated leukemia		After daunomycin
Author	Method	T½ in hours	T½ in hours
Killmann et al.	^{3}H Thymidine labeled blasts	23—22.5	
Clarkson et al.	^{3}H Uridine labeled blasts	28—32	
	^{3}H Thymidine labeled blasts	25—25	
Stryckmans et al.	^{3}H Cytidine labeled blasts	17.5	7—8—9—11

In untreated leukemia, within a few hours after an injection of ^{3}HTdr, labeled BM blasts are released into the blood [9]. This is illustrated on Fig. 2 (broken line) by the increase of the LI in the blood prior to the administration of Daunomycin. When Daunomycin was given immediately after ^{3}HTdr, i. e., while the labeled cells were still in the S phase, the output of labeled blasts from the BM to the blood was immediately blocked (solid lines Fig. 2). Theoretically when Daunomycin is injected 24 hours after ^{3}HTdr all the "flash" labeled cells should have the time to complete DNA synthesis ($\pm$20 hours) to pass G2 (3 hours) [10] and to enter G_1. When ^{3}HTdr and Daunomycin were injected according to this schedule (broken line Fig. 2), labeled cells could still be released from the BM to the blood after the injection of Daunomycin. This would indicate a preferential effect of the drug on the DNA synthesizing BM blasts. Whether this effect is cytostatic, cytocidal or both was looked for in the BM. Before Daunomycin treatment, the LI of BM blasts increased within 24 hours as a consequence of cell division (broken line Fig. 3). Such an increase was not observed when Daunomycin was injected 1 hour after ^{3}HTdr. This can not be accounted for by an arrest of cell division for cell division was not completely blocked as demonstrated by the decrease of the mean grain count of the labeled blasts. The only explanation for the observed decrease of the LI in the BM would be a cytocital effect on the leukemic blasts.

It has been shown in several systems that the fraction of proliferating cells in a cell population is greater when the size of this population is still small [12, 13]. In acute leukemia the proliferating cells can be recognised from the non proliferating by their larger size [6, 7, 14, 15].

As shown on Fig. 4 initially unlabeled cells enlarge and enter the large size categories 24 to 48 hours after the injection of Daunomycin. Prior to Daunomycin, the blast nuclei in the BM, showed a bimodal distribution of their size. The large nuclei (which included all the "flash" labeled nuclei) represented 20% of the whole blast population. Forthy eight hours after Daunomycin a bimodal distribution persisted but the large nuclei represented approximately 40% of the population. This suggests that as a consequence of the cytocidal effect of the drug, non proliferating "dormant" blasts, had re-entered proliferation within 48 hours.

Summary

Daunomycin seems to act as a cytocidal agent on all the leukemic blasts wathever their proliferative activity is, but the cells in the DNA synthesis phase are more sensitive to its action. Arguments are presented for the re-entering of "dormant" blasts in cycle within a day or two after an injection of Daunomycin.

References

1. Bernard, J., Jacquillat, Cl., Weil, M., Lortholary, P.: Essai de traitement des leucémies aiguës lymphoblastiques et myéloblastiques par un antibiotique nouveau: la rubidomycine. Etude de 61 observations. Presse méd. **75**, 951 (1967).
2. Silvestrini, R., Di Marco, A., Di Marco S., Dasdia, T.: Azione della daunomicina sul metabolismo degli acidi nuclei di Cellule normali e neoplastiche coltivate in vitro. Tumori **49**, 399 (1963).
3. Theologides, A., Yarbo, S. W., Kennedy, B. J.: Daunomycin inhibition of DNA and RNA synthesis. Cancer **21**, 16 (1968).
4. Di Marco, A., Silvestrini, S., Di Marco, S., Dasdia, T.: Effect of the new cytotoxic Antibiotic daunomycin on nucleic acids and mitotic activity of HELA cells. J. Cell. Biol. **27**, 545—550 (1965).
5. Kim, J. H., Gelbard, A. S., Djordjevic, B., Kim, S. H., Perez, A. G.: Action of daunomycin on the nucleic acid metabolism and viability of Hela cells. Cancer Res. **28**, 2437—2442 (1968).
6. Mauer, A. M., Fischer, V.: Characteristics of cell proliferation in four patients with untreated acute leukemia. Blood **28**, 428 (1966).
7. Killmann, S. A.: Acute leukemia; the kinetics of leukemic blast cells in man. Series Haematologica I no. 3, 1968, p. 38.
8. — Proliferative activity of blast cells in leukemia and myelofibrosis. Acta med. scand. **178**, 263 (1965).
9. — Estimation of phases of the life cycle of leukemic cells from labeling in human beings in vivo with tritiated thymidine. Lab. Invest. **12**, 671 (1963).
10. Clarkson, B. T., Ohkita, T., Ota, Fried, J.: Studies of cellular proliferation in human leukemia. I. Estimation of growth rates of leukemic and normal hematopoietic cells in two adults with acute leukemia given single injection of tritiated thymidine. J. clin. Invest. **46**, 506 (1967).
11. Stryckmans, P.: Unpublished data.
12. Lala, P. K., Patt, H. M.: Cytokinetic analysis of tumor growth: Proc. nat. Acad. Sci. (Wash.) **56**, 1735 (1966).
13. Frindel, E., Malaise, E. P., Alpen, E., Tubiana, M.: Kinetics of cell proliferation of an experimental tumor. Cancer Res. **27**, 1122 (1967).
14. Gavosto, F., Pileri, A., Bachi, C., Pegoraro, L.: Proliferation and maturation defect in acute leukaemic cells. Nature (Lond.) **203**, 92 (1964).
15. Saunders, E. F., Lampkin, B. C., Mauer, A. M.: Variation of proliferative activity in leukemic cell population of patients with acute leukemia. J. clin. Invest. **46**, 1356 (1967).

B. Asparaginase

Clinical Evaluation and Future Prospects of Asparaginase [1]

J. H. Burchenal

Division of Applied Therapy,
Sloan-Kettering Institute for Cancer Research and the Department of Medicine,
Memorial Hospital for Cancer and Allied Diseases, New York, N. Y.

With 6 Figures

The original discovery of the antileukemic effects of guinea pig serum by Kidd [1] in 1953 and the subsequent biological and chemical studies on its active principle, L-asparaginase (A-ase), by many investigators including Broome [2], Mashburn and Wriston [3], and Old, Boyse et al. [4, 5] are well known. Following the preliminary clinical studies on A-ase reported by De Barros et al. [6], Dolowy et al. [7], Hill et al. [8], and Oettgen et al. [9], we have been evaluating the drug for the past 2 years [10, 11].

Our clinical experience with A-ase at Memorial Hospital consists of 366 patients (206 adults and 160 children) treated with a dosage varying from 5 IU/kg daily to 5000 IU/kg daily, in most cases for at least 28 days. Of these patients, 214 had acute leukemias, a few had chronic leukemias, and the rest had various types of solid tumors. Although the place of A-ase in the armamentarium of the clinical chemotherapist cannot be exactly defined at present, certain data are available from these studies.

Schwartz et al. [12] have shown that after a single intravenous injection, peak plasma levels of A-ase were seen at 30 minutes, were the same for both the Merck and Bayer preparations of A-ase, and approximated the theoretical distribution in plasma. The half life of the Merck product was about 22 hours, however, whereas the half life of that from Bayer was about 11 hours. Thus, after repeated daily administration, the plasma levels in adults of A-ase 24 hours after the previous injection of 1000 IU/kg averaged about 26 IU/ml with the Merck and about 9 IU/ml with the Bayer preparation. Somewhat lower levels were obtained in children with both preparations. A new chemically modified A-ase from Bayer has a half life in man similar to the Merck sample [13]. There is no evidence, however, from any of

[1] These studies were supported in part by National Cancer Institute Grants CA-08748 and CA-05826 and American Cancer Society Grant T-45.

Table 1. *L-Asparaginase. Acute lymphoblastic leukemia—children*

Dose (IU/kg/day)	Total adequate	Duration of remission (days)
10	13	145, 105, 61, 45, 40, 38, 15
200	12	247, 125, 104, 63, 62, 50, 39, 37, 28
200×28	10	104, 103, 70, 57, 52, 19
1000×28	21	57, 58, 63, 74, 99, 100+, 102, 122, 123, 146, 191, 260, 278+
5000×28	11	15, 18, 20, 44, 120+, 125+, 158
Total	67	
Second trial		
5000×28	7	115, 58, 25
In remission onset of Rx		
1000×28	5	332+, 275+, 152, 141, 108
5000×28	4	74, 47, 19

our therapeutic data that the maintained level is more important than the peak level achieved immediately after injection, nor that one preparation is in any way superior to the other.

Toxicity studies reported by Oettgen et al. [14] showed that fever was very common, particularly with the early preparations with a low specific activity per milligram protein, ranging from 87% with the early preparations to approximately 50% with the later preparations. There was weight loss in most of the cases at all dosage levels, but it appeared to be more severe at 5000 IU/kg per day. Lethargy and confusion were seen in about one-third of the children and somewhat more of the adults. Fall in serum cholesterol occurred in most patients, and was followed in two patients by a very marked increase in cholesterol and triglycerides. Some decreases in serum albumin levels were seen in most of the patients, but only in rare cases did they go below 50% of the pretreatment level. In most patients there was an increase in levels of IgM, IgA, and IgG. Abnormality in liver function tests was common, with elevated SGOT, increased BSP retention, and the fall in albumin levels being the most common evidence of impaired liver function. There was an increase of BUN, associated with A-ase therapy, in 34% of children and over 80% of adults. Approximately a third of the patients had hypersensitivity reactions associated with the first course of A-ase therapy, but over two-thirds had a serum antibody to the particular enzyme preparation used [14].

A-ase will produce remissions in patients with acute lymphoblastic leukemia, whether children or adults, in about 50 to 70% of the patients [15, 16]. The incidence of remission seems to be approximately the same regardless of the dose from 10 to 5000 IU/kg, as can be seen from Table 1. Seven out of 13 remissions were achieved at 10 IU/kg, 6 out of 10 at 200 IU/kg, 13 out of 21 at 1000 IU/kg, and 7 out of 11 at 5000 IU/kg. Although the groups are small and somewhat inhomogeneous, there does, however, seem to be some advantage of a dosage level of 1000 IU/kg for 28 days, as compared to 200 IU/kg daily for 28 days, in the duration of remission, as shown in

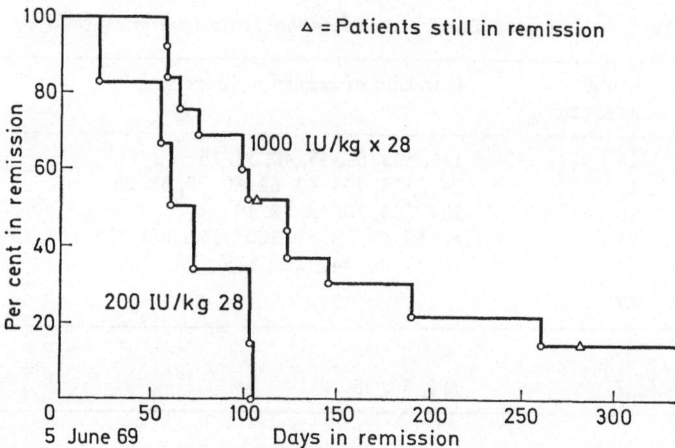

Fig. 1. Effect of dose of asparaginase on length of unmaintained remission in acute lymphoblastic leukemia in children

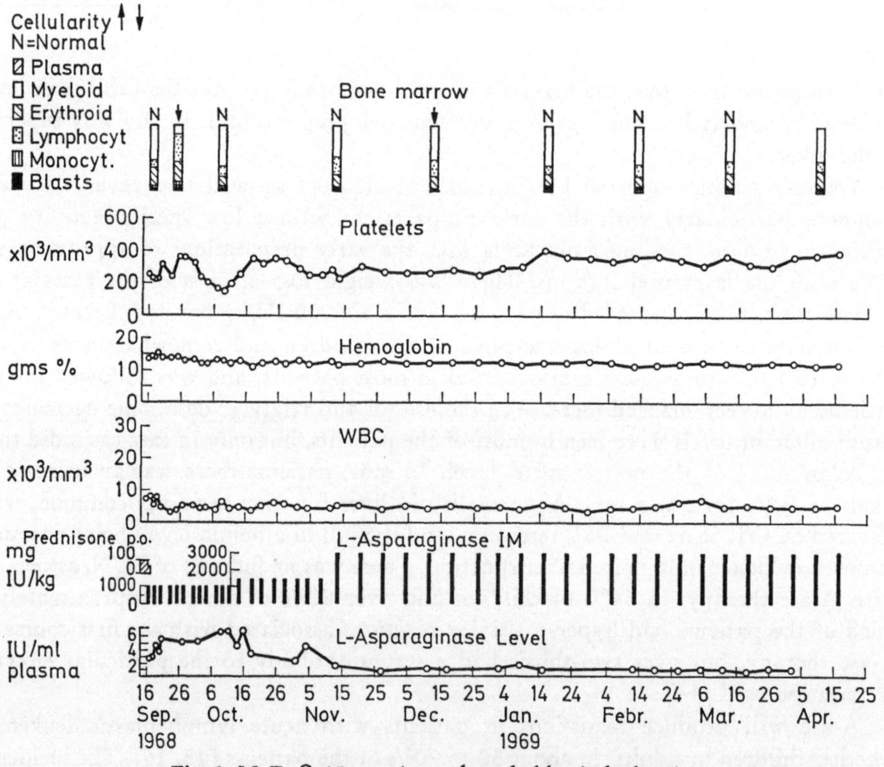

Fig. 2. M. F. ♀ 15 yrs. Acute lymphoblastic leukemia

Table 1 and in Fig. 1. The intramuscular use of the drug was also tried, and in one patient given once weekly doses of 3000 IU/kg for 7 months (Fig. 2), plasma levels of A-ase taken before each weekly injection showed approximately 0.8 IU/ml [12]. The patient finally relapsed after a total of almost 9 months of therapy.

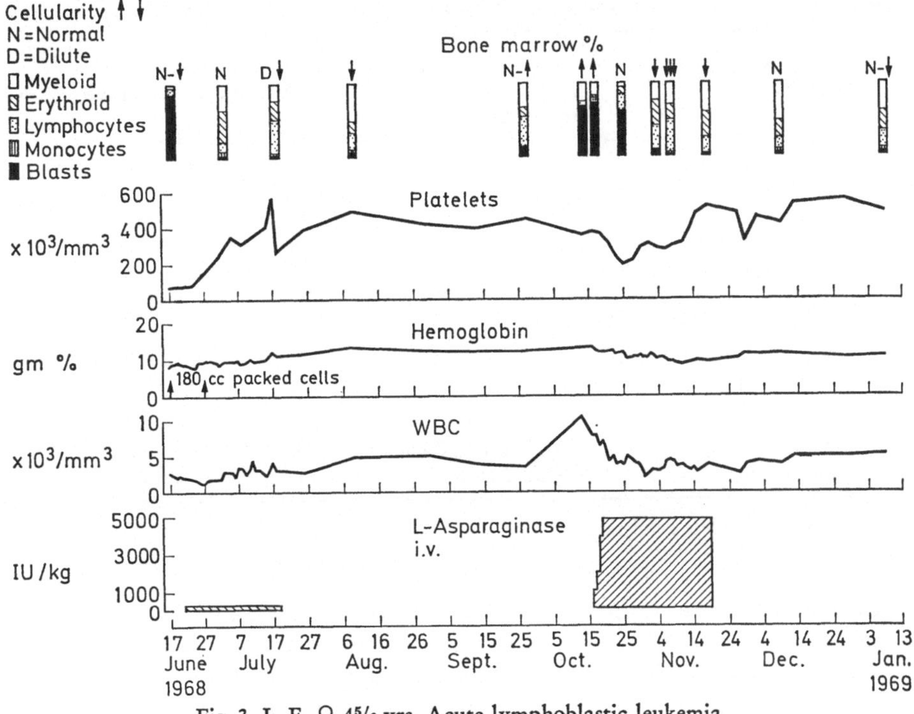

Fig. 3. L. E. ♀ 4 5/6 yrs. Acute lymphoblastic leukemia

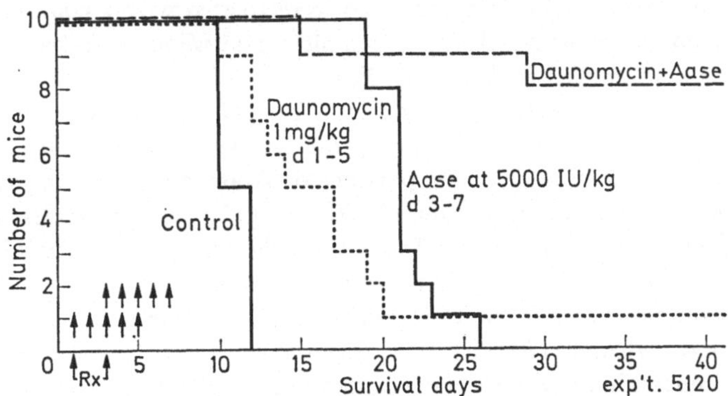

Fig. 4. Effect of Daunomycin and A-ase on leukemia L5178Y I. P.

In acute myeloblastic leukemia in adults, complete or good partial remissions have been achieved in 4 of 32 patients (12%). In many other cases, however, there has been a fall in white count and some decrease in nodes, liver, or spleen during the first week of therapy, only to relapse while under continued therapy. This suggests that these leukemic cells are initially dependent on asparagine but have the capability of inducing the enzyme, asparagine synthetase, very rapidly in the absence of asparagine.

Over 150 adults [16] and children [15] with solid tumors have been treated with A-ase, but with the exception of rare temporary remissions in lymphomas and in one case of melanoma, we have seen no beneficial effects in any of the solid tumors.

Table 2. *Inhibition of incorporation of ^{3}H-valine into protein in vivo by cells of mouse and human leukemias in absence of asparagine and presence of A-ase*

Leukemia	*In vivo* sensitivity	Percentage inhibition −Asparagine	+A-ase
Mouse leukemia:			
EARAD1	S	57	75
L5178Y	S	39	78
L5178Y/CA55	S	53	86
EARAD1/A-ase	R	0	8
L5178Y/CA55/A-ase	R	2	7
L1210	R	0	0
P815	R	5	0
Human A. L. L.:			
E. F.	S (CR [a] 4 mo.)	24	41
L. E.	S (CR 3 mo., 3 mo.)	7	25
M. K.	S (CR 5 mo.)	12	23

[a] CR = complete remission

The development of resistance to A-ase has been relatively rapid, and some of the patients have relapsed on continued therapy as little as 2 weeks after the remission was induced. Others have relapsed only after 8 months of continuous therapy. One is still in unmaintained remission 9+ months after a 28-day course of A-ase 1000 IU/kg. In none of the patients who relapsed while on maintenance therapy were we able to induce a second remission. In 7 patients who were treated with a course of A-ase for 28 days with no maintenance therapy, complete remissions on a second course of therapy were again achieved in three (Fig. 3).

A test based on the work of Sobin and Kidd [17], which uses the relative inhibition of incorporation of ^{3}H-valine into protein, in leukemic cells incubated *in vivo* in the absence of asparagine or in the presence of A-ase, to predict the sensitivity to A-ase *in vivo*, is very accurate in mouse leukemias [18] but is much less satisfactory in human leukemias, as can be seen in Table 2. Further modifications will be necessary to make this a useful predictive test in the human disease.

Studies in mouse leukemia have demonstrated that prior treatment with 1-β-D-arabinofuranosyl cytosine (Ara-C) and thioguanine [19] (Table 3) in leukemia EARAD1, or concomitant therapy with Daunomycin [18] (Fig. 4) or vincristine [18] (Fig. 5) in the somewhat less sensitive leukemia L5178Y, produces much better results, particularly in regard to 50-day cures, than either member of the combination alone. Fig. 6 shows a child with acute leukemia in whom a remission was induced with vincristine and prednisone and consolidated with Ara-C and thioguanine for 28 days, followed by 1000 IU/kg of A-ase daily for 28 days in May and June 1968. She has been on no maintenance since July 1968 and is still in complete remission as of June 1969.

At the present time we are treating patients with a combination of A-ase, 30,000 IU/m^2 i.v. daily for 28 days; prednisone, 60 mg/m^2 p.o. daily for 28 days; vincristine, 1.5 to 2.0 mg/m^2 i.v. once weekly for 4 doses; and Daunomycin, 45 mg/m^2 i.v. on days 15, 17, and 19. At the end of the 28-day period, these patients are given

Table 3. *Effect of prior treatment with Ara-C and TG*[a] *on antileukemic activity of a single dose of A-ase against leukemia EARAD1 i. p.*

Compound	Dose[b]	wt. day 12	Survival time	% ILS[c]	50 day survival
Control		−0.4	14.4		
A-ase	500	−1.4	26.6	+ 85	
Ara-C	10	+0.5	24.3	+ 68	
TG	0.5	−0.6	14.3	− 1	
Ara-C TG	10 0.5	−0.5	27.5	+ 90	1
Ara-C A-ase	10 500	−1.0	46.7	+224	7
TG A-ase	0.5 500	−1.1	40.8	+183	3
Ara-C TG A-ase	10 0.5 500	−0.1	50.0	+247	10

[a] TG = thioguanine
[b] Ara-C and TG given in mg/kg daily days 3 through 7. A-ase given in international units/kg as a single dose on day 7.
[c] ILS = increase in life span

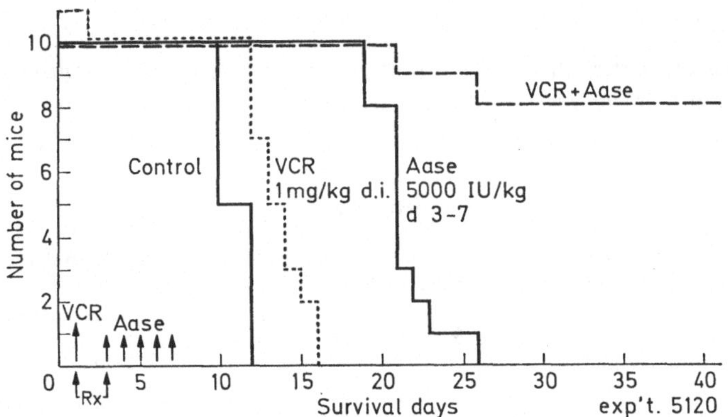

Fig. 5. Effect of vincristine (VCR) and A-ase on leukemia L5178Y I. P.

no maintenance therapy and are observed for length of remission. A very high incidence of initial remissions with considerable evidence of increased toxicity has been observed so far, but it is too early to assess the duration of unmaintained remissions. In the acute myeloblastic leukemia, A-ase 1000 IU/kg i.v. daily for 28 days is combined with Ara-C, 3 mg/kg i.v. and thioguanine, 2.5 mg/kg p.o. daily for 5 or more doses, to the point of mild leukopenia. Again the A-ase appears to enhance the marrow toxicity of Ara-C and thioguanine, and care should be taken to avoid undue marrow depression.

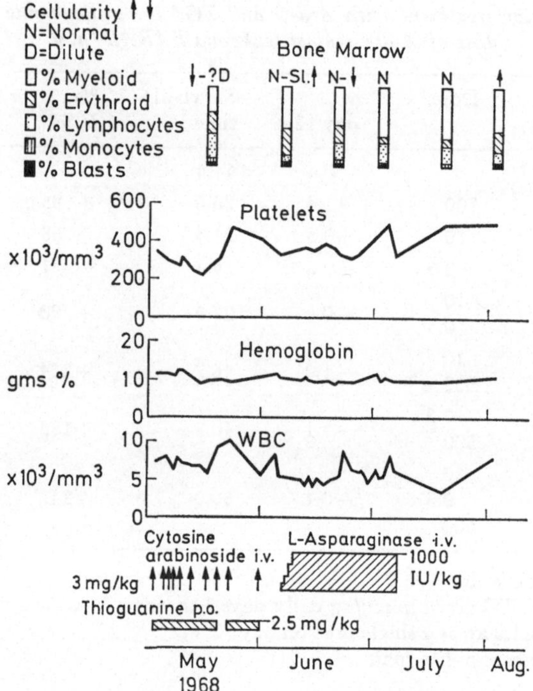

Fig. 6. D. I. ♀ 3¹/₁₂ yrs. Acute lymphoblastic leukemia

In conclusion, although the exact place of A-ase in clinical chemotherapy of acute leukemia cannot be defined at present, it is hoped by such combination therapy to increase the total leukemic cell kill and thus achieve prolonged remissions.

Summary

L-asparaginase has been shown to be active against many types of animal lymphomas and leukemia, and against acute lymphoblastic leukemia, and to a lesser extent acute myeloblastic leukemia in patients. Its activity in mouse leukemias is markedly potentiated by cytosine arabinoside, Daunomycin, or vincristine. Although the exact place of asparaginase in clinical chemotherapy of acute leukemia cannot be defined at present, it is hoped by such combination therapy to increase the total leukemic cell kill and thus achieve prolonged remissions.

References

1. Kidd, J. G.: Regression of transplanted lymphomas induced in vivo by means of normal guinea pig serum. I. Course of transplanted cancers of various kinds in mice and rats given guinea pig serum, horse serum, or rabbit serum. J. exp. Med. **98**, 565—581 (1953).
2. Broome, J. D.: Evidence that the L-asparaginase of guinea pig serum is responsible for its antilymphoma effects. I. Properties of the L-asparaginase of guinea pig serum in relation to those of the antilymphoma substance. J. exp. Med. **118**, 99—120 (1963).
3. Mashburn, L. T., Wriston, J. C.: Tumor inhibitory effect of L-asparaginase from Escherichia coli. Arch. Biochem. Biophys. **105**, 450—452 (1964).
4. Old, L. J., Boyse, E. A., Campbell, H. A., Daria, G. M.: Leukaemia-inhibiting properties and L-asparaginase activity of sera from certain South American rodents. Nature (Lond.) **198**, 801 (1963).

5. Boyse, E. A., Old, L. J., Campbell, H. A., Mashburn, L. T.: Suppression of murine leukemias by L-asparaginase. Incidence of sensitivity among leukemias of various types: comparative inhibitory activities of guinea pig serum L-asparaginase and Escherichia coli L-asparaginase. J. exp. Med. **125**, 17—31 (1967).
6. De Barros, T., Filho, M. C., De Santana, C. F., Valenca, M., Da Silva, M. P., Guedes, J., De Carvalho, A. R. L.: Utilizacao de L-asparaginase em paciente humano portador de neoplasia maligna. An. Fac. Med. Recife **25**, 21—28 (1965).
7. Dolowy, W. C., Henson, D., Cornet, J., Sellin, H.: Toxic and antineoplastic effects of L-asparaginase. Cancer **19**, 1813—1819 (1966).
8. Hill, J. M., Roberts, J., Loeb, E., Kahn, A., MacLellan, A., Hill, R. W.: L-asparaginase therapy for leukemia and other malignant neoplasms. J. Amer. med. Ass. **202**, 882—888 (1967).
9. Oettgen, H. F. et al.: Inhibition of leukemias in man by L-asparaginase. Cancer Res. **27**, 2619—2631 (1967).
10. Burchenal, J. H., Oettgen, H. F.: The present clinical status of asparaginase. UICC (Union Internationale Contre le Cancer) Bulletin **7**, 5 (1969).
11. — Karnofsky, D. A., Murphy, M. L., Oettgen, H. F.: Effects of L-asparaginase on leukemias and other neoplasms. International Society of Hematology, XIIth Congress (New York 1968), Abstracts of the Simultaneous Sessions, p. 7.
12. Schwartz, M. K., Lash, E. D., Oettgen, H. F., Tomao, F. A.: L-asparaginase activity in plasma and other biological fluids. Cancer Feb. 1970.
13. Haberland, G.: Personal communication.
14. Oettgen, H. F., Stephenson, P. A., Schwartz, M. K., Leeper, R. D., Tallal, L., Clarkson, B. D., Golbey, R. B., Krakoff, I. H., Karnofsky, D. A., Burchenal, J. H.: The toxicity of *E. coli* L-asparaginase in man. Cancer Feb. 1970.
15. Tallal, L., Tan, C., Oettgen, H., Wollner, N., McCarthy, M., Helson, L., Burchenal, J., Karnofsky, D., Murphy, M. L.: E. coli L-asparaginase in the treatment of leukemia and solid tumors in 131 children. Cancer Feb. 1970.
16. Clarkson, B., Krakoff, I., Burchenal, J., Karnofsky, D., Golbey, R., Oettgen, H., Dowling, M., Lipton, A.: Clinical results of treatment with E. coli L-asparaginase in adults with leukemia, lymphoma, and solid tumors. Cancer Feb. 1970.
17. Sobin, L. H., Kidd, J. G.: A metabolic difference between two lines of lymphoma 6C3HED cells in relation to asparagine. Proc. Soc. exp. Biol. Med. (N. Y.) **119**, 325—327 (1965).
18. Burchenal, J. H.: Success and failure in present chemotherapy and the implications of Asparaginase. Proceedings of the ACS-UICC Conference, "A Ccritical Evaluation of Cancer Chemotherapy" (Cherry Hill, N. J. 1969). Cancer Res. Dec. 1969.
19. — Dollinger, M. R.: L-asparaginase in transplanted mouse leukemia. International Society of Hematology, XIIth Congress (New York 1968), Abstracts of the Simultaneous Sessions, p. 6.

The Place of the L-Asparaginase in the Treatment of Acute Leukemias

G. Mathé, J. L. Amiel, A. Clarysse, M. Hayat, and L. Schwarzenberg

Institut de Cancérologie et d'Immunogénétique, Hôpital Paul-Brousse 14, Avenue Paul-Vaillant-Couturier, 94-Villejuif
et Service d'Hématologie de l'Institut Gustave Roussy 16 bis, Avenue Paul-Vaillant-Couturier, 94-Villejuif, France

With 3 Figures

L-asparaginase has, in a few months, taken an important place in the chemotherapy of leukaemias, its clinical utilisation has confirmed the interest in the drug (Mathé et al., 1969), defined its indications and also its limits; it has made it possible to discover that the enzyme was not without action on normal cells; we shall report the results obtained at Villejuif, and dwell on certain secondary effects, which were not pointed out by the first users (Burchenal et al., 1968; Hill et al., 1967).

Methods and Patients

Methods

L-asparaginase is administered intravenously at the rate of two daily injections. The doses are varied from 400 U./kg/day to 1000 U./kg/day, i. e. 32.000 U./m²/day. The total dose is not fixed in advance, it is either the maximum tolerated dose, or a dose sufficient to obtain an optimal effect, or determined by the objective signs of resistance to the treatment.

Patients

We have carried out 135 courses of treatment with L-asparaginase, on 130 patients. The ages of the patients varied from 1 to 62 years. The distribution of the patients is indicated in Table 1.

Therapeutical Results

In acute lymphocytic leukaemias in the visible phase, the results are shown in Table 2.

Table 1. *Patients treated by L-asparaginase*

				Number of patients	No. of courses of treatment
Acute lymphoblastic leukaemia	In visible phase	Treated by L-asparaginase alone		28	31
		Treatment by L-asparaginase combination with prednisone, vincristine and rubidomycin		12	12
	In non-visible phase	Treated by asparaginase alone	Not in hypoplastic phase	31	31
			In hypoplastic phase	13	13
		Treated by L-asparaginase in combination with methotrexate		11	11
Acute myeloblastic leukaemia	In visible phase	Treated by L-asparaginase alone		3	5
		Treated by L-asparaginase in combination with prednisone, vincristine and rubidomycin		10	10
Blastic crises	Of chronic myelocytic leukaemia			5	5
	Of polycythemia vera			1	1
	Of lymphoblastosarcoma			4	4
Melanosarcomas				12	12
				130	135

Table 2. *L-asparaginase given alone in the treatment of visible phases of acute lymphoblastic leukaemia*

Patients	Courses of treatment	Complete remissions
28	31	12 [a]

[a] 3 in 2nd visible phase. 6 in 3rd visible phase, 1 in 6th visible phase, 1 in 9th visible phase. 1 in 10th visible phase.

Out of 31 courses of treatment on 28 patients, we have obtained 12 complete remissions (i. e. 43%). These remissions can occur very late in the evolution of the disease, 3 in 2nd phase, 6 in 3rd phase, 1 in 6th phase, 1 in 9th phase, 1 in 10th phase.

L-asparaginase was used in association with prednisone, vincristine and rubidomycin in 12 cases of acute lymphocytic leukaemia, which had previously been shown to be resistant to the association of prednisone-vincristine, with 6 complete remissions here again in late phase of the disease, 4 in 2nd phase, 1 in 3rd phase, 1 in 4th phase of the disease (Table 3).

In acute myeloblastic leukaemia (Table 4) with L-asparaginase alone we treated 3 patients one of them being a baby of 8 months; this baby had 3 successive courses

Table 3. *L-asparaginase given in combination with prednisone (40 mg/m²/d), vincristine (1,5 mg/m²/week) and rubidomycin (30 mg/m²/twice a week in child; 10 mg/m²/twice a week in adult) in acute lymphoblastic leukaemia after a failure of prednisone + vincristine*

Patients	Courses of treatment	Complete remissions
12	12	6[a]

[a] 4 in 2nd visible phase. 1 in 3rd visible phase. 1 in 4th visible phase.

Table 4. *L-asparaginase in the treatment of acute myeloblastic leukaemia*

	Patients	Courses of treatment	Complete remissions
L-asparaginase alone	3	5[a]	3[b]
L-asparaginase given in combination with prednisone, vincristine and rubidomycin	10	10	2

[a] 3 for a 8 months old baby. [b] 2 for a 8 months old baby.

Table 5. *L-asparaginase given in combination with prednisone, vincristine and rubidomycin in the treatment of blastic crises in chronic myelocytic leukaemia, polycythemia vera and lymphoblastosarcoma*

		Patients	Courses of treatment	Complete remissions
Blastic crises in	Chronic myelocytic leukaemia	5	5	1
	Polycythemia vera	1	1	
	Lymphoblastosarcoma	4	4	3

of treatment with 2 successes and finally a failure, we obtained a second complete remission on a 3rd phase of the disease in an adult.

In combination with prednisone, vincristine and rubidomycin, we treated 10 patients with 2 complete remissions in the 1st phase of the disease.

We have used L-asparaginase in association with prednisone, vincristine and rubidomycin in 10 cases of transformation into acute leukaemias, and we have obtained a complete remission in one case of acute transformation of chronic myelocytic leukaemia out of 5 and in 3 cases of transformation of lymphoblastosarcoma out of 4 (Table 5).

The total failure of L-asparaginase in melanosarcoma must be pointed out: 12 cases, 12 total failures. L-asparaginase was given in association with vincristine and methotrexate.

Secondary Effects and Complications of L-asparaginase

We have been able to study them in favourable conditions as we have given L-asparaginase alone in 44 cases of acute lymphoblastic leukaemias in the non-visible phase of their disease; in 31 cases the differential blood count being pratically normal at the beginning of the course of L-asparaginase, in 13 cases the patients were in hypoplastic state at the beginning of this treatment (less than 1000 polynuclear cells/mm^3), which detered us from following the antimitotic treatment.

1. Tolerance of the Product

In 8 cases we have recorded the appearance of an anaphylactic reaction (Table 6). In 4 of these cases the anaphylactic reaction appeared during an attempt to restart a treatment, by L-asparaginase after a period without treatment, in 2 cases the reaction appeared during the first treatment by the product after tolerating well 14 and 17 daily injections respectively.

Table 6. *Anaphylactic reactions to asparaginase*

Courses of treatment	Anaphylactic reaction		
	To a second course of treatment	During a first course of treatment	To a first injection of asparaginase
130	4	2	2

In two cases we have observed a reaction of the anaphylactic type during the *first* injection of L-asparaginase. In one of these cases the patient had a past history of severe infantile asthma.

We have made 3 attempts of desensitization without success.

We have frequently noticed nauseas, once continued fever which fell when the product was stopped.

The important point to us seems to be that the appearance of an anaphylactic reaction, obliges to give up all hope of restarting the treatment.

2. Effects on Hematopoiesis

The group of patients treated by L-asparaginase alone in the non-visible phase of the disease allows to assess in a valid manner the effect of the product on hematopoiesis.

a) In 31 patients having normal blood counts at the beginning of the treatment, there was no alteration of the Hb; we did not see anemias as others have reported. There was a slight decrease in platelet count, but not in a significant degree. Much more striking was the progressive decrease in total white cell count and the absolute neutrophil count. This was a constant finding. In spite of some marked neutropenias we did not have any infectious complications.

b) 13 patients were neutropenic before the beginning of the treatment (median 1410 granulocytes/mm^3).

It is important to point out that if L-asparaginase can induce a neutropenia, it does not aggravate a pre-existing neutropenia to complete aplasia, as can be seen on Table 7.

After treatment by L-asparaginase alone the median granulocytic count was 1430. Overall there was little change; most patients remained leukopenic, but they

Table 7. *Haematological studies during L-asparaginase therapy 10 days L-asparaginase in 31 cases in remission*

	Median	
	Before	After
Hemoglobin	13.8	14.1
Platelets	195,000	145,000
White blood cells	7,850	3,600
Absolute P. M. N. count	5,150	1,540

Table 8. *L-asparaginase during chemotherapy induced neutropenia*

	Number of cases	Median granulocytic count	
		Before treatment	After treatment
L-asparaginase alone	8	1410	1430
L-asparaginase + prednisone	5	1380	2050

did not become more leukopenic and there were actually 5 patients in whom the neutrophil count increased slightly; there were patients that received prednisone simultaneously with L-asparaginase. Here again we did not have any infectious complications. Thus it seems that L-asparaginase can be safely used in spite of its neutropenia producing effect, even in leukopenic patients (Table 8).

3. Effects on the Hepatic Functions and Particularly on Hemostasis (Table 9)

The study was done on 70 patients receiving L-asparaginase alone.

The most significant point is the fall of fibrine level; it is almost constant; beside all visible phase of the disease. The other factors of hemostasis are affected in a much less constant way (Fig. 1).

Table 9. *Biochemistry during L-asparaginase treatment given alone in 70 patients*

	Median		
	Before	After	
Urea	0.32	0.42	g ‰
Cholesterol	1.97	1.93	g ‰
Alk. phosphatases	10	13	K. A. U.
Bilirub. total	5.3	6.8	mg ‰
S. G. P. T.	40	62	F. U.
S. G. O. T.	20	44	F. U.
O. C. T.	424	488	i. u.
Total serum proteins	64	57	g ‰
Albumin	34.8	28.6	g ‰
Fibrine	3.98	1.8	g ‰

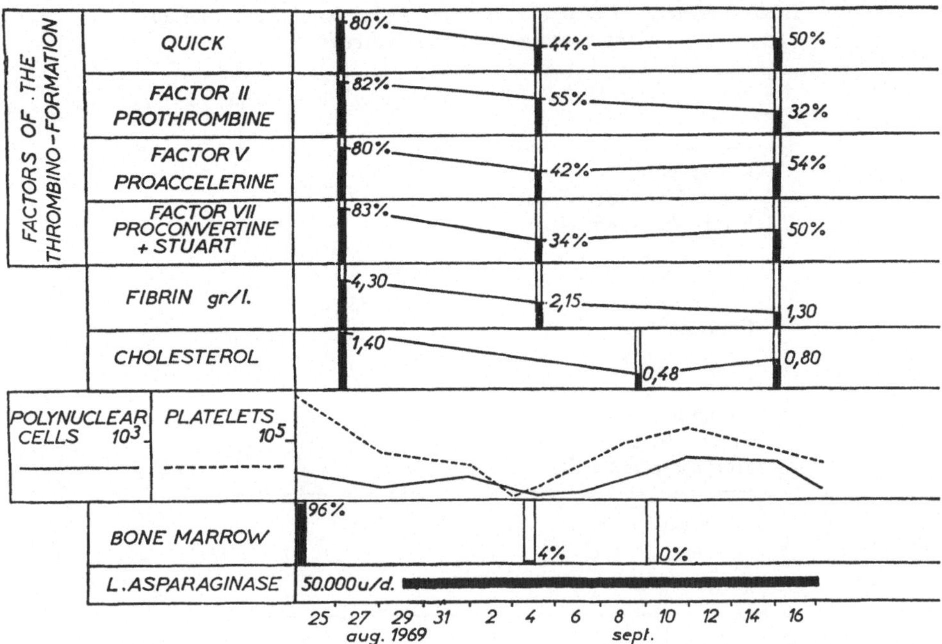

Fig. 1. Effect of L-asparaginase on various factors of the hepatic function and hemostasis

The other hepatic factors are little or not disturbed. In our studies, there is a slight and inconstant decrease of albumin, cholesterol stays usually normal; we have noted a case of severe hypocholesterolemia; the cholesterol level fell from 1.40 g at the beginning of treatment to 0.48 g/l after 15 days of L-asparaginase 50,000 U/day.

4. Effects on the Immunological Functions

These are difficult to evaluate directly in Man, even in cases of treatment of subjects in non-visible phase of their leukaemia; in fact, the treatment by L-asparaginase succeeds immunosuppressive antimitotic treatments and the comparison of results obtained before and after treatment by L-asparaginase have therefore little significance.

We have therefore conducted a study in Mouse within the framework of the trial programmes of the E.O.R.T.C.

a) Effects on the Reaction to Sheep Red Cells

18 (DBA/2×C57Bl/6) F1 female adult mice are randomised in three groups of 6 mice: A, B, C. Each mouse receives peritoneally on day 0, 10^9 sheep red cells; on day 5, the spleens are removed and the number of plaque forming cells in gelified solution is determined for each spleen (Jerne and Nordin, 1963).

The mice in group A receive on days —3, —2 and —1, and those in group B on days 1, 2 and 3, 100 units of L-asparaginase intraperitoneally per mouse and per day.

The results are summed up in Table 10.

Table 10. *Effects of L-asparaginase on the immunological reactions of mice against sheep red cells*

	Mean number of plaque forming splenic cells
Group A Treated by asparaginase before sheep red cells	14,900
	S for P < 0.02
Group C Controls	43,700
	NS
Group B Treated by asparaginase after sheep red cells	41,700

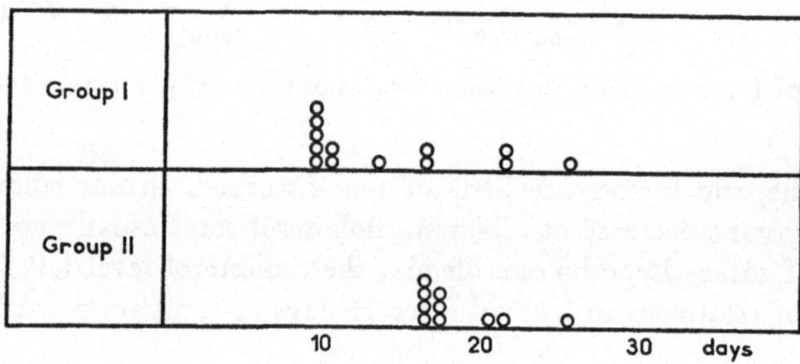

Fig. 2. Effect of L-asparaginase on graft-versus-host reaction. F1(DBA/2×C57Bl/6) mice irradiated (500 rads) receiving 10^7 bone marrow cells and 2.5×10^7 lymph node cells from C57Bl/6 donors

Group I: not treated donors. Group II: donors treated by L-asparaginase

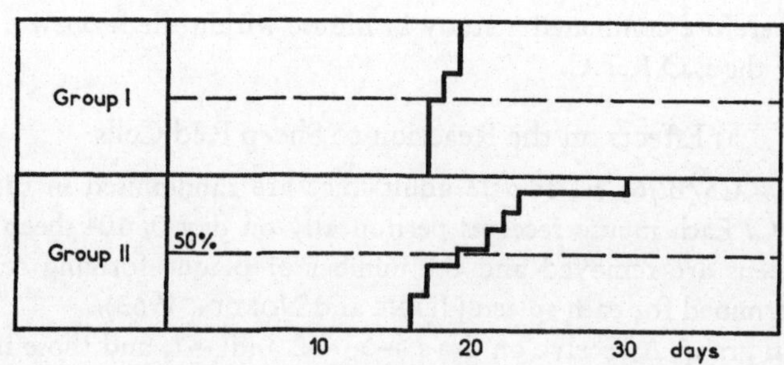

Fig. 3. Effect of L-asparaginase on allogeneic skin graft tolerance. Recipients CBA. Donors C57Br

Group I: not treated recipients. Group II: recipients pretreated by L-asparaginase

L-asparaginase given before the antigenic stimulus depresses the immunological reaction in a manner statistically valid, while given after the antigenic stimulus it is without action.

b) Effects on the Graft-Versus-Host Reaction

23 mice F1(DBA/2×C57Bl/6) are totally irradiated at day 0 at the dose of 500 rads. They are randomized in two groups. 13 mice of group I receives I.V., at day 0 after irradiation, 10^7 bone marrow cells and 2.5×10^7 lymph node cells of adult C57Bl/6 donors. 10 mice of group II receive the same number of cells but from donors pretreated on days —3, —2, —1, by L-asparaginase, 100 Units/mice/day, I. P.

The mean survival time in the group I is 14.6 days and in the group II 19.1 days (S for $P < 0.05$).

c) Effects on Allogeneic Skin Grafts

15 mice CBA ($H—2^k$) are randomized in two groups. 6 mice of group I are not treated; 9 mice of group II received on days —3, —2, —1, 100 Units/mice/day, of L-asparaginase I. P. On day 0, every mice receives a skin graft of C57Br donors ($H—2^k$). The mean survival time of the graft in the first group is 16.3 days and in the second group 19.7 days. The comparison by the non parametric test w of Wilcoxon shows that the difference is significant.

These results are in good correlation with these of Hobik (1969) showing some immunosuppressive effect of L-asparaginase on the graft-versus-host reaction in rat and mice, and with these of Ohno (1969) showing an inhibition of lymphocyte blastogenesis by PHA in vitro by L-asparaginase.

In conclusion our experience allows us to clear several points.

1) L-asparaginase can induce complete remissions in acute lymphoblastic leukaemias at a very late stage of the disease, and resistant to most other chemotherapies.

In our experience these remissions were obtained in 12 treatments out of 31, or about 40 p. 100.

2) L-asparaginase has a certain leukopenia producing effect, but hardly aggravates the pre-existing leukopenia by its use. It can therefore be used during complementary chemotherapy of acute leukaemias in non-visible phases during these periods of hypoplasia.

3) L-asparaginase does not seem to us, used in association with prednisone, vincristine and rubidomycin in the visible phases of acute leukaemias, with methotrexate in non-visible phases, to add appreciably to the toxicity due to antimitotics. It can therefore be integrated in the schemes of chemotherapies of acute leukemias.

4) L-asparaginase frequently induces an immunisation manifested by anaphylactic shocks, the most often during the 2nd or 3nd course of treatment, sometimes during the first course of treatment, and sometimes from the first injection. These anaphylactic shocks must be distinguished from incidents of the type of anorexia, nauseas, fever; they entail the stopping of the treatment; the attempts of desensitization were not efficient in our experience.

5) L-asparaginase is not without effect on the hepatic functions, a marked decrease of fibrin is observed very frequently; but we were led to stop the treatment due to the hepatic toxicity only once.

6) L-asparaginase is immunosuppressive, as least in the animal; it can not, therefore be used at the same time as an active immunotherapy (AMIEL and BERARDET, 1969).

Summary

1) L-asparaginase can induce complete remissions in acute lymphoblastic leukaemias at a very late stage of the disease, and resistant to most other chemotherapies.

In our experience these remissions were obtained in 12 treatments out of 31, or about 40 p. 100.

2) L-asparaginase has a certain leukopenia producing effect, but hardly aggravates the pre-existing leukopenia by its use. It can therefore be used during complementary chemotherapy of acute leukemias in non-visible phases during these periods of hypoplasia.

3) L-asparaginase does not seem to us, used in association with prednisone, vincristine and rubidomycin in the visible phases of acute leukemias, with methotrexate in non-visible phases, to add appreciably to the toxicity due to antimitotics. It can therefore be integrated in the schemes of chemotherapies of acute leukemias.

4) L-asparaginase frequently induces an immunisation manifested by anaphylactic shocks, the most often during the 2nd or 3rd course of treatment, sometimes during the first course of treatment, and sometimes from the first injection. These anaphylactic shocks must be distinguished from incidents of the type of anorexia, nauseas, fever; they entail the stopping of the treatment; the attempts of desensitization were not efficient in our experience.

5) L-asparaginase is not without effect on the hepatic functions, a marked decrease of fibrin is observed very frequently.

6) L-asparaginase is immunosuppressive, as least in the animal; it cannot, therefore, be used at the same time as an active immunotherapy.

References

AMIEL, J. L., BERARDET, M.: Essai de traitement de la leucémie E ♂ G 2 associant chimiothérapie et immunothérapies actives spécifique ou non spécifique. Rev. franç. Étud. clin. biol. 14, 685 (1969).

BURCHENAL, J. H., KARNOFSKY, D. A., MURPHY, M. L., OETTGEN, H. F.: Effects of L-asparaginase on leukemia and other neoplasms. In.: C. R. XIIe Cong. Int. Soc. Hematol., 1 vol. New York 1968, p. 7.

HILL, J. M., ROBERTS, J., LOEB, E., KHAN, A., HAYTON, M., HILL, R. W.: L-asparaginase therapy for leukaemia and other malignant neoplasms. J. Amer. med. Ass. 202, 882 (1967).

HOPIK, H. P.: Immunosuppressive Wirkung von L-asparaginase in der Graft-versus-Reaktion. Naturwissenschaften 56, 217 (1969).

JERNE, N. K., NORDIN, A. A., HENRY, C. C.: The agar plaque technique for recognizing antibody producing cells. In: Cell bound antibodies. Philadelphia: Wistar Institute Press 1963, p. 109.

MATHÉ, G., AMIEL, J. L., SCHWARZENBERG, L., SCHNEIDER, M., CATTAN, A., SCHLUMBERGER, J. R., HAYAT, M., DE VASSAL, F., JASMIN, C., ROSENFELD, C.: Essai de traitement de la leucémie aigue lymphoblastique par la L-asparaginase. Presse méd. 77, 461 (1969).

OHNO, R.: Inhibition of lymphocyte blastogenesis by L-asparaginase. Proc. Amer. Ass. Cancer Res. 10, Abstr. 261 (1969).

Clinical Experience with L-Asparaginase in Britain

G. Hamilton Fairley

Chester Beatty Research Institute, Royal Marsden Hospital, Sutton, Surrey
and St. Bartholomew's Hospital, London

With 2 Figures

So far in Britain we have had three sources of l-asparaginase, two obtained from *E. coli* (supplied by E. R. Squibb and Farbenfabriken Bayer A.G.) and one from *Erwinia carotovorum* (Microbiological Research Establishment in Britain). The supplies have been distributed by the Medical Research Council and used principally at The Hospital for Sick Children, Great Ormond Street, by Professor Hardisty, and at the Royal Marsden Hospital and St. Bartholomew's Hospital by Dr. Galton and myself.

Supplies from Squibb were small and, therefore, most of our experience so far has been with the material supplied by Bayer. Our overall results in acute leukaemia are very similar to those described by Burchenal and his collagues at this symposium. Of the 65 patients with acute lymphoblastic leukaemia treated so far, we have obtained complete remissions in one-third of the patients, partial remissions in another third and no response in the remainder. With acute myeloblastic leukaemia there have been no complete remissions when the drug was used alone but some effect was observed, the significance of which will be discussed.

Administration and Toxicity

The dose used has been between 200 and 1000 IU/kg/day given by twice daily intravenous injection; and because we know that the enzyme is virtually confined to the plasma (J. G. Hall, 1969, personal communication) we now use a dose based on surface area (35,000 IU/M^2/day).

We have observed the usual toxicity of nausea and vomiting, a fall in the blood levels of fibrinogen and albumen, and slight abnormalities in liver function tests. We have not encountered pancreatitis as described by Schein et al. (1969) and this may be due to the fact that the Bayer l-asparaginase is obtained from *E. coli* A, whereas the Merck material used by Schein et al. (1969) is obtained from *E. coli* B. Indeed, this raises the important point that whenever the toxicity or the efficacy of l-asparaginase is discussed, it is essential to know which material is being used, as there are significant differences between the rate of clearance and toxicity of the enzyme from different sources.

Hypersensitivity has developed in several of our patients, and can prove troublesome. In two patients once hypersensitivity occurred we changed to using Porton l-asparaginase, and confirmed the experimental work at Porton that there is no cross-sensitivity between the *E. coli* and *Erwinia* enzymes. Indeed, antibodies raised against the *E. coli* enzyme do not cross-react with those raised against *Erwinia*. (A. P. MACLENNON, 1969, personal communication). Clearly to have a second source of enzyme which is antigenically completely different may prove to be very useful.

Clinical Response in Acute Leukaemia

In acute lymphoblastic leukaemia the speed of clinical response to Bayer l-asparaginase shows considerable variation. In some cases the blast cells are removed very rapidly from the blood although the effect on the bone-marrow may occur very much later. An example of this is shown in Fig. 1 a. A girl aged 6 with acute lymphoblastic leukaemia who had previously received prednisone, vincristine, methotrexate and cyclophosphamide was given l-asparaginase and within 72 hours the blast cell count in the peripheral blood fell from 250,000/cu mm to zero. However, the bone-marrow still contained blast cells after 21 days of treatment, but at the end of the course (i. e. 28 days) these had disappeared and a complete remission was obtained. During this period intra-thecal methotrexate had to be given for cerebral leukaemia, but the blood had been cleared of leukaemic cells before methotrexate was used. This patient has been treated subsequently with l-asparaginase. The second course once again produced rapid clearance of blast cells from the peripheral blood, and a slower return of the marrow to normal (Fig. 1 b). The third course acted initially in the same way but on the 17th day of treatment blast cells appeared again in the blood and rose rapidly, so that treatment with l-asparaginase was stopped (Fig. 1 c). However, when the leukaemic cells were tested 20 days later for their sensitivity to the drug *in vitro* using the technique of OETTGEN et al. (1967) the cells still showed sensitivity to the action of the enzyme; after 18 hours incubation there was a reduction of 60% in the uptake of tritiated uridine by the cells grown in a medium free from asparagine or with added asparaginase, when compared with the uptake in the medium containing asparaginase.

In acute myeloblastic leukaemia no complete remissions have been obtained, but in three patients there was a marked effect on the number of circulating leukaemic cells. This is illustrated in Fig. 2 which shows the effect of l-asparaginase on the peripheral blood of a man aged 60 with acute myeloblastic leukaemia. The blast count initially was 143,000/cu mm and the *in vitro* test showed that the cells were sensitive to the enzyme. After treatment for 8 days the blast count fell to 1300/cu mm but slowly rose again to reach 54,000/cu mm after 19 days. At this time the cells were not sensitive to the action of the enzyme *in vitro*. Cytosine arabinoside was used and only after the third course did leukaemic cells disappear from the blood. A similar effect has been seen in two other patients. For this reason we feel that l-asparaginase may have a useful role in reducing the number of leukaemic cells but should be used in combination with other anti-leukaemic drugs such as cytosine arabinoside and 6-mercaptopurine.

Professor HARDISTY has had considerable success in treating children with lymphoblastic leukaemia with cytosine arabinoside followed by l-asparaginase, and in the

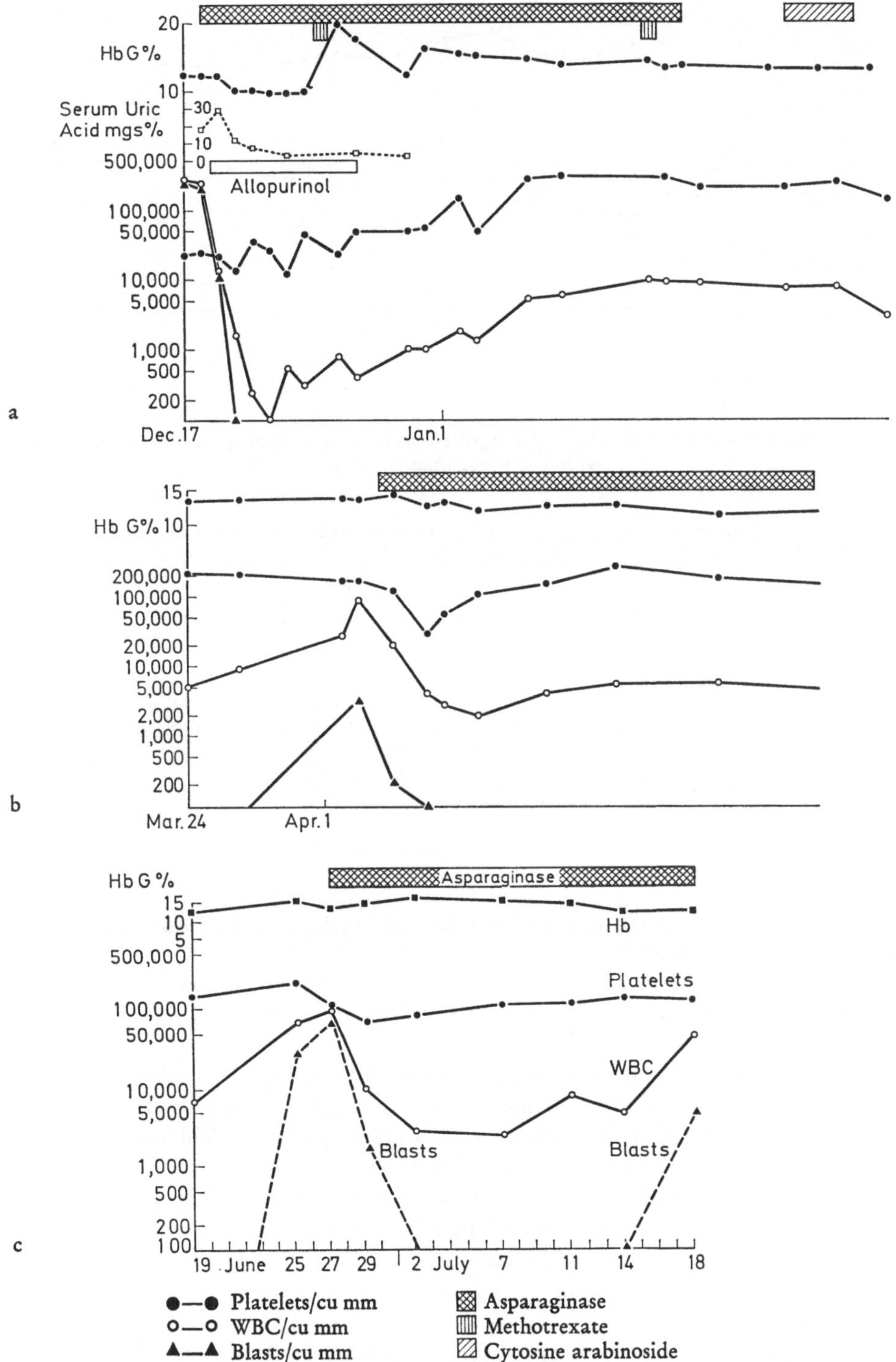

Fig. 1. Peripheral blood changes in a child aged 6 with acute lymphablastic leukaemia (a) during the first, (b) the second and (c) the third course of L-asparaginase (Bayer)

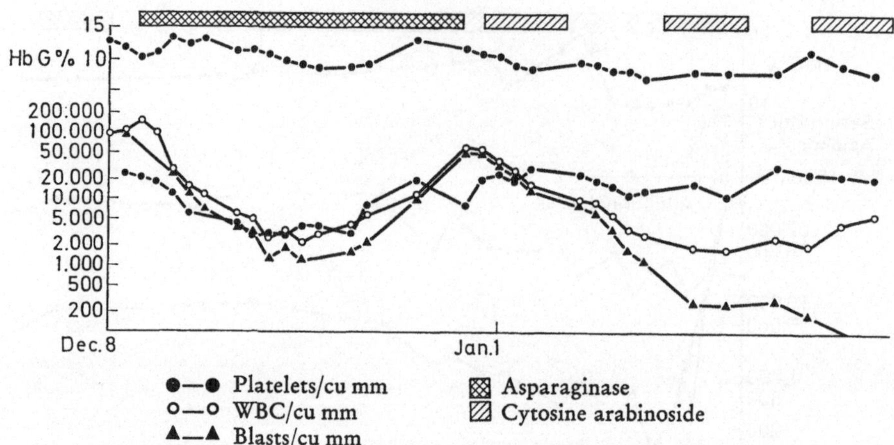

Fig. 2. Peripheral blood changes in a man aged 60 with acute myeloblastic leukaemia treated with L-asparaginase (Bayer)

Table 1. *Cytotoxic effect of L-asparaginase on malignant melanoma cells in vitro*

Number of cases	Concentration of asparaginase in I.U./ml			
	0	10	20	40
5	0	+	+	+
4	0	0	+	+
5	0	0	0	+
15	0	0	0	0
Total 29				

future almost certainly the enzyme will be best used in combination with other agents in this disease as well.

The development of resistance to the action of l-asparaginase has been disappointing and has limited its usefulness in the treatment of leukaemia. There are several possible explanations.

First, it is possible from the outset that there are two populations of cells, one of which is sensitive, and the other resistant. Secondly, depriving the cells of asparagine may induce the formation of the enzyme asparagine synthetase. Thirdly, it is possible that where blast cells exist in close proximity to normal cells, there could be direct feeding of asparaginase by the normal cells. Such a mechanism might explain the fact that blast cells may be removed rapidly from the blood, where the cells are floating freely in an environment containing asparaginase, but only slowly from the marrow where the interstitial fluid contains very little asparaginase and the cells are tightly packed.

We have recently become interested in l-asparaginase in malignant melanoma in view of the one patient who has responded to treatment with this drug at The Memorial Hospital, New York (Burchenal, 1969, personal communication). We have had no clinical success using this drug in malignant melanoma, but growing the melanoma cells in tissue culture in Pulvertaft chambers Dr. MARTIN LEWIS has found that the concentration required to kill the cells is very variable. Table 1 summarises our results. In 15 cases the addition of l-asparaginase to the culture medium (TC. 199) had no effect but in the remaining 14 cases a cytotoxic effect was observed although in 5 cases as much as 40 IU/ml was required to achieve this. It may be that this cytotoxic effect is due to the glutaminase present both in *E. coli* and *Erwinia* asparaginase, since melanoma cells survive in Pulvertaft chambers in TC. 199 which does not contain asparagine.

Summary

L-asparaginase is already a useful agent in the treatment of acute lymphoblastic leukaemia, and may be of some benefit in acute myeloblastic leukaemia particularly if used in combination with other drugs.

Great care must be taken to state exactly which asparaginase is concerned in any report, as the blood levels and toxic effects vary depending on the source of the enzyme.

L-asparaginase obtained from *Erwinia carotovorum* is completely different antigeneically from *E. coli* and if hypersensitivity to *E. coli* material occurs, the *Erwinia* enzyme can be used with safety.

The problem of leukaemic cells becoming resistant to the action of the drug, and the role of glutaminase require further investigation.

References

OETTGEN, H. F., OLD, L. J., BOYSE, E. A., CAMPBELL, H. A., PHILIPS, F. S., CLARKSON, B. D., TALLAL, LISA, LEEPER, R. D., SCHWARTZ, M. K., KIM, J. H.: Inhibition of leukemias in man by L-asparaginase. Cancer Res. **27**, Pt. 1, 2619—2631 (1967).

SCHEIN, P. S., RAKIETEN, N., GORDON, B. M., DAVIS, RUTH D., RALL, D. P.: The toxicity of Escherichia coli L-asparaginase. Cancer Res. **29**, 426—434 (1969).

Clinical Status of L-Asparaginase and Side Effects

C. G. Schmidt, W. M. Gallmeier, and H. W. Stier

Innere Klinik und Poliklinik (Tumorforschung) der Ruhruniversität, Klinikum Essen

The first attempts to use asparaginase in patients were reported by De Barros in 1965 [2] and by Dolowy et al. in 1966 [4]. These investigators used enzyme-containing fractions of the sera of agoutis and guinea pigs respectively. They noted a slight antitumor effect in one case of melanoma and one case of acute lymphoblastic leukemia. Complete remissions of acute lymphoblastic leukemia in patients treated with E. coli asparaginase were first reported by Hill et al. [7] and Oettgen et al. in 1967 [10].

After one year of clinical trials with l-asparaginase in Europe and even a longer period of intensive clinical investigation of this drug in the USA, it's usefulness as well as it's limitation are becoming quite clear. There was hardly a drug with so great a discrepancy between expected side effects and toxicity actually seen. Although it could be shown that l-asparaginase worked by a completely different mechanism than all other chemotherapeutic agents so far used it had been found that the range of asparaginase sensitive malignancies is almost exclusively confined to certain leukemias [10, 12].

To select sensitive patients we initially employed the in-vitro test as prescribed by Oettgen et al. [10, 13]. Although we recorded a generally good correlation between the results of this test and the initial clinical response we later learned, that this initial favorable response is by no means a parameter for the ultimate remission or failure of treatment [5]. We no longer use this test as a routine screening method.

As in other reports [10, 12] encouraging results were seen in patients with acute lymphoblastic leukemias. We treated 8 patients with the standard dose of 200 IU/kg body weight. 6 patients went into remission, 4 of them had a complete remission with less than 5% blasts in their marrow count. One patient, a 24 year old young man who received the standard treatment of 200 IU/kg over a period of 4 weeks is now in remission for more than 18 month without any maintenance therapy, his performance status is excellent, he is working again.

Since this manuscript, was accepted for publication a relapse of the ALL occured. The new established leukemic cell line does no longer belong to the asparaginase-sensitive population. The repetition of the predictive test revealed a negative result corresponding very well with a high level of asparaginase-synthetase measured too.

Of the 11 patients with acute non lymphoblastic leukemias, all had had previously multiple courses of chemotherapy. All but one responded with initially favorable objective signs such as significant fall in peripheral leukemic cells, rise of serum uric acid, decrease of the spleen size etc. Invariably however the bone marrow remainded unchanged and the number of leukemic cells in the periphery increased again. There was no influence on the ultimate course of the disease, even if the dose of asparaginase was increased to 1000 IU/kg or more.

We treated 6 patients with chronic myelocytic leukemia of the ones who reacted positive in vitro. All presented the signs of an initial favorable response, but only 2 went into remission which could be maintained by further treatment with busulfan. It may be of interest that patients with osteomyelofibrosis also react favorably when treated with l-asparaginase: The number of immature cells in the peripheral blood decreased and the spleen size became normal.

Since only 2 out of 15 patients with chronic lymphatic leukemia were sensitive in vitro, we only treated these. The size of the spleen and the lymphnodes became normal, the peripheral cell count however rose considerably. Finally resistance developed and other chemotherapy had to be employed.

Inspite of clearcut positive in vitro tests no significant response was seen in patients with myelomas and malignant melanomas. There was no response in patients with other lymphomas, or solid tumors.

The greatest rate of response is with patients with acute lymphoblastic leukemia but even here, as reported by Burchenal and others [1 a], the percentage of complete remissions is lower than can be obtained with one of the modern combination regimens in spite of the fact that asparaginase does offer a new approach to the treatment of acute lymphoblastic leukemias. On the other hand Asparaginase does not offer anything new in the treatment of acute non lymphoblastic leukemias and the chronic myelogenous or lymphatic leukemias.

The side effects and toxicity by far exceed the ones which had been anticipated from the theoretical point of view i. e. the mode of action of this drug and the experience from the drug in experimental animals [10]. These side effects have been milder in children than in adults. As in reports from other Centers [9, 10] we have seen chills, fever (at high doses), nausea, loss of appetite and weight, lethargy and other mental changes, allergic reactions and precipitating antibodies against the asparaginase preparation, changes in serum lipids such as decrease of the cholesterol level, decrease of serum proteins such as the alpha-2-globulin fraction, increase of the serum enzymes such as GOT, GPT, 5-Nukleotidase, alkaline phosphatase and bilirubin, rise of the BUN values. We have not recorded diabetes or disturbances in the pancreatic function. The hematologic side effects included thrombopenia, anemia and sometimes leukopenia.

We have been particularly interested in the disturbances of the clotting system and studied the clotting factors fibrinogen, prothrombin, accelerator globulin (V), proconvertin (VII) and antihaemophilic globulin (VIII) and generally found that the concentration of all these factors decreased several days after the beginning of asparaginase administration [14]. These disorders not only occurred in patients with asparaginase sensitive leukemias but also in patients with asparaginase resistant tumors and were found in normal rabbits too. Concerning the low activity of asparagine synthetase in normal liver tissue [8] these findings are thought to be in some extent caused by a significant reduction of the protein-synthesis due to a fall of asparagine in the liver and the reticulo-endothelial-system. This point of view is supported by the clinical finding that asparaginase disturbs the liver function as mentioned above.

Furthermore in several cases of acute leukemia and chronic myelogenous leukemia a subacute consumption-coagulopathy intensifying the defribination could be demonstrated by a fall of thrombocytes and a slight fibrinolysis. Consistant with this interpretation DEUTSCH [3] found a decrease of the plasminogen concentration in the treated leukemic subjects. At present time the fibrinogen degradation products in the blood of treated persons are being examined in our laboratory.

HASKELL et al. [6] demonstrated fibrinogen split products in the blood of a patient with renal failure during the therapy indicating intravascular coagulation. This disorder mostly occurred in patients with considerable induced cell destruction. The liberation of thromboplastic substances from the destroyed leukemic cells can be discussed as the pathogenetic factor. The transitory hyperuricemia in these patients may have a supporting role in triggering the activation of the intravascular coagulation. A generalized SANARELLI-SCHWARTZMAN-reaction by a contamination with E. coli endotoxin of the asparaginase preparation used could be excluded by animal experiments. As shown by means of the thrombelastography and the fibrin-plate-method L-asparaginase does not influence the coagulation of normal blood in vitro. A clear cut effect of heparin application on this disorder could seldom be seen. This may be due to the superimposed inhibition of clotting factor synthesis. Furthermore the anti-heparin activity of leukemic cells [1 b] may be involved. In instances where we have not observed the expected rise in thrombocytes after heparin application this could be due to the advanced leukemic state of the patients. We dot not know on the other hand if asparaginase in addition effects the rate of proliferation of megakaryocytes in leukemic bone marrow. By a simple incubation experiment with normal citrated blood we could exclude the possibility that asparaginase directly destroys the platelets. The plasmatic clotting defects seldom required substitution. The limiting factor in certain circumstances is the thrombopenia induced by the treatment with l-asparaginase. This condition requires careful precautions. We lost one patient by an untreatable bleeding.

Although l-asparaginase is not the first choice of treatment in patients with acute lymphoblastic leukemia, we have seen complete remissions in such patients in whom conventional chemotherapy has been exhausted. This fact and the possible role of l-asparaginase in combination with other agents warrants it's further use and study.

Summary

6 out of 8 patients with acute lymphoblastic leukemia, treated with a standard dose of 200 IU/kg/day went into remission. 4 had a complete remission, one of these patients has been in remission for more than 18 months now without any maintenance therapy. In 11 patients with acute non-lymphoblastic leukemia there was no effect on the ultimate course of the disease, although some objective responses were seen in 10 patients. 2 patients with chronic lymphocytic as well as chronic myelogenous leukemia responded initially but resistance developed under treatment. The side effects of this treatment include fever, nausea, weight loss, lethargy, allergic reactions, changes in serum lipids, elevation of the transaminases, thrombopenia and anemia. These reactions only rarely require treatment to be stopped. Furthermore there are abnormalities of the clotting system, which are due to deficient synthesis of the clotting factors in the liver and RES. In some cases we observed a subacute consumption coagulopathy, also induced by the enzyme treatment. L-asparaginase is a useful drug for the treatment of acute lymphoblastic leukemias, where it brings about remissions in cases where all chemotherapy has been exhausted. Its use in combination with other drugs remains to be evaluated.

References

1 a. Burchenal, J. H., Karnofsky, D. A., Murphy, M. L., Oettgen, H.F.: Effects of L-Asparaginase on Leukemias and other Neoplasms. XIIth Congress. International Soc. Hemat. New York 1968.

1 b. Cacciola, E., Ferranto, A.: Presence of antiheparin in activity in leukemic cells. Boll. Soc. ital. Sper. **36**, 1317 (1968).

2. De Barros, T.: Utilizacao de L-Asparagina em patiente humano portador de neoplasia maligna. An. Fac. Med. Recife **25**, 21 (1965).

3. Deutsch, E.: Discussion at the Internationale Arbeitstagung über Chemo- und Immuntherapie der Leukosen und malignen Lymphome. Wien/Austria, March 1969.

4. Dolowy, W. C., Henson, D., Cornet, J., Sellin, H.: Toxic and antinoplastic effects of L-asparaginase. Cancer **19**, 1813 (1966).

5. Gallmeier, W. M., Schmidt, C. G., Stier, H. W.: In-vitro-Testung von Zellen auf Asparaginmangelempfindlichkeit in Chemo- und Immunotherapie der Leukosen und malignen Lymphome. Hrsg. A. Stacher. Wien: Bohmann Verlag 1969, p. 30.

6. Haskell, C. M., Canellos, G. P., Leventhal, B. G., Carbone, P. P., Serpick, A. A., Hansen, H. H.: L-asparaginase toxicity. Cancer Res. **29**, 974 (1969).

7. Hill, J. M., Roberts, J., Loeb, E., Khan, A., McLettan, A., Hill, R. W.: L-asparaginase therapy for leukemia and other malignant neoplasma. J. Amer. med. Ass. **202**, 882 (1967).

8. Horowitz, B., Madras, B. K., Meister, A., Old, J. J., Boyse, E. A., Stockert, E.: Asparagin synthetase activity of mouse leukemias. Science **160**, 533 (1968).

9. Mathé, G., Amiel, J. L., Schwarzenberger, L., Schneider, M., Cattan, A., Schlumberger, J. R., Hayat, M., de Vassal, F., Jasmin, J., Rosenfeld, S.: Essai de traitement de la leucémie aigue lymphoblastique par la L-asparaginase. Presse méd. **77**, 461 (1965).

10. Oettgen, H. F., Old, L. J., Boyse, E. A., Campbell, H. A., Philips, F. S., Clarkson, B. D., Talal, L., Leeper, K. D., Schwartz, M. K.: Inhibition of leukemias in man by L-asparaginase. Cancer Res. **27**, 2619 (1967).

11. Oettgen, H. F., Schulten, H. K.: Hemmung maligner Neoplasien des Menschen durch L-Asparaginase. Klin. Wschr. **47**, 65 (1969).

12. Oettgen, H. F.: Paper presented at the meeting of the Paul-Ehrlich-Gesellschaft Wuppertal — Asparaginase-Therapie der Leukämien. May 1969.

13. Schmidt, C. G., Gallmeier, W.: Zur Enzymtherapie der Leukämien. Dtsch. med. Wschr. **93**, 2299 (1968).

14. Stier, H. W., Schmidt, C. G., Gallmeier, W. M.: Das Blutgerinnungssystem während der Leukämiebehandlung mit L-Asparaginase in Chemo- und Immuntherapie der Leukosen und malignen Lymphome. Hrsg.: A. Stacher. Wien: Bohmann Verlag 1969, p. 310.

Asparaginase: Early Clinical and Toxicology Studies

P. P. Carbone, C. M. Haskell, G. P. Canellos, B. G. Leventhal, J. Block, A. A. Serpick, and O. S. Selawry

Medicine Branch, National Cancer Institute Bethesda, Maryland, and Baltimore Cancer Research, Baltimore, Maryland

Asparaginase represents the first successful application of a biochemical enzyme to cancer therapy [1, 2]. The destruction of asparagine by systemic administration of asparaginase kills tumor cells that are dependent on asparagine and have an impaired ability to synthesize asparagine. At the NCI, 55 patients have received 50 to 2000 IU/kg/day of *E. coli* l-asparaginase. The present report summarizes the clinical and toxicologic effects using the Merck, Sharp, and Dohme (MSD) or Squibb and Company (SC) preparation.

Study Plan

E. coli l-asparaginase (NSC-109229) was obtained from SC as a soluble powder with varying degrees of specific activity of 121—231 IU/mg protein and from MSD as 321—363 IU/mg protein. The enzyme was administered in 0.9% saline or 5% dextrose over a 30 to 40 minute period. Twenty-four patients with various solid tumors and 31 patients with leukemia received the drug. All except 6 patients had received prior therapies. Antitumor response was evaluated by $\geqq 25\%$ decrease in measurable disease or standard evaluation of leukemia status [3].

All patients were skin tested and were found to be non-reactive. They received 50 to 2000 IU/kg by daily infusion, with 2/3 of the patients receiving 200 IU/kg/day usually for 3 weeks.

Results

In the solid tumor patients responses were seen in one of 5 patients with malignant melanoma and one complete and 3 partial responses ($\geqq 50\%$) in seven patients with malignant lymphosarcoma. Complete marrow remissions were seen in one of 6 patients with acute myelocytic leukemia and 2 of 8 adults with ALL. In children with ALL 3 of 11 patients had complete remissions. The remissions unmaintained were 2 toweeks and with various maintenance schedules 5 to 27 weeks.

The major forms of drug toxicity are summarized in Table 1. Drug related toxicity was defined as an abnormality which did not exist prior to treatment and appeared after treatment. The most common forms of toxicities were nausea and

Table 1. *L-asparaginase toxicity*

Problem	Patients evaluable	Patients with problem	Patients with serious problem
Nausea, Anorexia, Vomiting	50	33	6
Fever	44	30	5
Hypersensitivity	55	14	9
Anemia	8	5	0
Clotting Abnormalities	20	16	1
Liver Dysfunction	35	33	4
Azotemia	35	17	2
Pancreatitis	54	6	3
CNS—Adults Only	35	18	5

vomiting with anorexia and fever of $> 1°$ C above baseline. Hypersensitivity manifested itself as urticaria most frequently, but 5 patients had respiratory embarrassment, one developed hypotension, and one a severe serum sickness-like reaction. A decrease in hemoglobin of $\geqq 2$ g-%o occurred in 5 of 8 evaluable patients. In the patients with solid tumors, no leukopenia or thrombocytopenia was documented. Clotting test abnormalities occurred in 16 of 20 patients with evaluable studies. These included depression of plasma fibrinogen, prolonged prothrombin and partial thromboplast in time.

Liver function disturbances were noted in 33 of 35 evaluable patients usually expressed as a decrease in albumin or cholesterol or increase in alkaline phosphatase or bromsuphalein retention. Fatty infiltration of the liver was seen on biopsy in 2 patients. Azotemia, defined as an increase in blood urea nitrogen (BUN) above 20 mg-%o, occurred in 17 to 35 patients, usually clearly interpretable as a pre-renal problem. However, 2 patients had oliguria and markedly elevated BUNs. One had evidence for intravascular clotting and the other developed hyperglycemia, hypovolemia and acute tubular necrosis.

Pancreatitis was a major and unexpected finding in 6 patients. The pancreatitis occurred with as little as 3 days of asparaginase treatment. Another unusual toxic reaction was central nervous system dysfunction noted in 18 of 35 patients. In 4 patients severe confusion and disorientation occurred with abnormal electroencephalograms noted in 2 patients, and a fifth patient developed a severe emotional depression. These reactions occurred from the 19th to the 31st day at 200 IU/kg, 17 days at 400 IU/kg, and 5 days at the 1500 IU/kg level.

Discussion

Asparaginase represents a unique agent with clear cut activity in lymphocytic neoplasms, particularly ALL [2, 4]. The optimal schedules of administration and dosage level are not as yet defined. The serum half-life of asparaginase is in the order of 12 to 18 hours with these preparations. Yet the persistent absence of asparagine from the serum for 4 to 7 days after therapy is discontinued implies an active storage site in the body, possibly in the reticuloendothelial system that continues to destroy asparagine. At the dosages administered above the levels of asparaginase achieved are 10 to 100 times higher than necessary to eliminate circulating asparagine. What the important aspect of chemical attack is, be it the dissipation of serum asparagine, the depletion of total body asparagine stores, or the levels of asparaginase for deamidation of other biologic substances, remains to be answered.

Regarding toxicity, asparaginase therapy, while sparing the bone marrow, obviously affects the liver, kidney, pancreas, and brain [5]. Since it is a foreign protein, *E. coli* asparaginase acts as an antigen resulting in immunologic side effects. In addition asparaginase contains small amounts of endotoxin with its attendant side effects. The cause of some of the side effects may be related to asparaginase's unique property of shutting off protein synthesis, i. e. serum proteins [6], clotting factors [7], and insulin [8]. Other side effects are undoubtedly related to contaminants [9] or deamidation of other substrates [10]. Crystalline asparaginase will soon be available for clinical trials to help answer some of these questions.

Summary

L-asparaginase was administered to 24 patients with solid tumors and 31 patients with acute leukemia at doses of 50 to 2000 IU/kg daily for one to three weeks. The manifestations of drug induced toxicity included fever, nausea, hypersensitivity reactions, and liver function disturbances. However, major life threatening toxicity occurred infrequently and was related to pancreatitis, renal failure and central nervous system depression occurring in about 15% of patients. Significant tumor responses were seen in patients with acute lymphocytic leukemia and lymphosarcoma.

References

1. Broome, J. D.: Studies on the mechanism of tumor inhibition by L-asparaginase. J. exp. Med. **127**, 1055—1072 (1968).
2. Oettgen, H. F., Old, L. J., Boyse, E. A., Campbell, H. A., Philips, F. S., Clarkson, B. D., Tallal, L., Leeper, R. D., Schwartz, M. K., Kim, J. H.: Inhibition of leukemias by L-asparaginase. Cancer Res. **27**, (Part 1) 2619—2631 (1967).
3. Bisel, H. F.: Criteria for the evaluation of response to treatment in acute leukemia. Blood **11**, 676—677 (1956).
4. Hill, J. M., Roberts, J., Loeb, E., Khan, A., MacLellan, A., Hill, R. W.: L-asparaginase therapy for leukemia and other malignant neoplasms. J. Amer. med. Ass. **202**, 882—888 (1967).
5. Haskell, C. M., Canellos, G. P., Leventhal, B. G., Carbone, P. P., Serpick, A. A., Hansen, H. H.: Letter to the editor: L-asparaginase toxicity. Cancer Res. **29**, 974—975 (1969).
6. Canellos, G. P., Haskell, C. M., Arseneau, J., Carbone, P. P.: Hypoalbuminemic and hypocholesterolemic effect of L-asparaginase (NSC-109229) treatment in man: preliminary report. Cancer Chemother. Rep. **53**, 67—69 (1969).
7. Gralnick, H. R., Henry, P. H.: L-asparaginase induced coagulopathy. Proc. Amer. Ass. Cancer Res. **10**,32 (1969).
8. Whitecar, J. P., Jr., Harris, J. E., Bodey, G. P., Freireich, E. J.: Host effects of L-asparaginase treatment. Clinical Res. **17**, 408 (1969).
9. Zweifach, B. W., Janoff, A.: Bacterial endotoxemia. Ann. Rev. Med. **16**, 201—202 (1965).
10. Cooney, D. A., Handschumacher, R. E.: Investigation of L-asparagine metabolism in animals and human subjects. Proc. Amer. Ass. Cancer Res. **9**, 15 (1968).

Preliminary Results of L-Asparaginase in Acute Leukemias

M. Weil, C. Jacquillat, M. Boiron, and J. Bernard

Institut de Recherches sur les leucémies, Hôpital Saint-Louis, Paris

With 1 Figure

We shall report briefly the results obtained with L-asparaginase in our Department Hopital St. Louis.

We have so far treated 84 patients with L-asparaginase, but in 9 patients treatment was undertaken at a terminal stage of disease and death occurred before the results could be evaluated. We shall thus consider the results obtained in 75 patients. 40 patients were treated with L-asparaginase alone, and 35 patients with a combination including L-asparaginase. Distribution of patients is shown on Table 1.

Table 1. *Distribution of patients*

	Asparaginase alone	Combination	Total
A. L. L.	34	27	61
A. M. L.	6	8	14
Total	40	35	75

A. Results in A. L. L. of L-asparaginase Given Alone

Daily doses in A. L. L. were generally 1000 units per kg. Results are reported in Table 2; they were better in first attacks (6/11 complete remissions) than in relapses (7/23 complete remissions). In our experience, disappearance of blast cells was rapid in blood, more progressive in bone marrow. Complete aplasia, the median duration of which was 10 days, was observed in some cases.

The median day of complete remission was 15.

In two cases, one of which is shown in Fig. 1, the complete remission of meningeal relapses was observed with systemic L-asparaginase, while in two other cases a meningeal blastosis appeared in the course of maintenance treatment with L-asparaginase; this maintenance treatment consisting in biweekly intramuscular doses of L-asparaginase was given to 6 patients in A. L. L.

The median duration of remissions was 3.5 months.

Table 2. *Results with L-asparaginase in the treatment of A.L.L. related to the phase of disease*

	1st attack	1st relapse	2nd relapse	3rd relapse	4th relapse	Total
Complete remissions	5+1[a]	2	3	2	0	12+1[a]
Partial remissions	0	2	0	1	0	3
Partial failure	4	1	2	0	0	7
Total failure	0	2	4	2	2	10
Death on treatment	1[a]+1[b]					1[a]+1[b]
Total	11	7	9	5	2	34

[a] Death on day 30 in a patient in C. R. having had a total colectomy for multiple perforations on day 20.

[b] Death on day 6 by intracranial bleeding.

June 1969

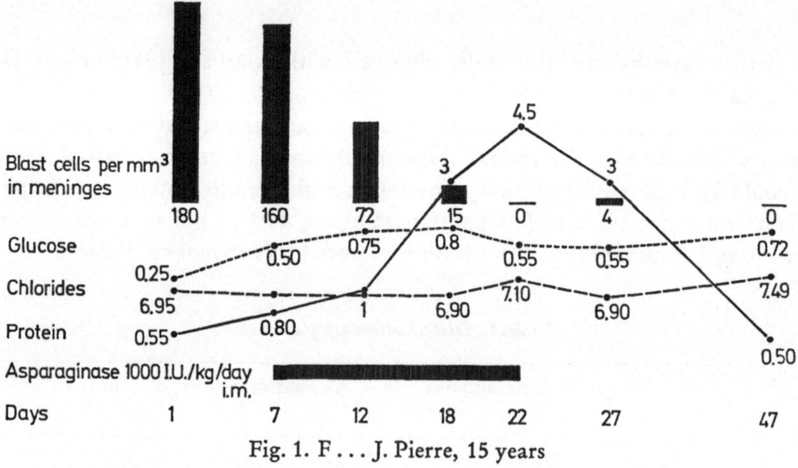

Fig. 1. F . . . J. Pierre, 15 years

B. Results in A. M. L. of Asparaginase Given Alone

In A. M. L. daily doses were 4000 units per kg. Results are shown in Table 3.

In 2 out of 6 cases complete remissions were noted in 2 children; in these patients no granulation was seen with May-Grunwald Giemsa stains but cytochemical study detected small peroxidase-positive granulations.

Table 3. *A. M. L. treated by L-asparaginase alone (4000 i. u./kg/day)*

	1st attack	1st relapse	2nd relapse	Total
C. R.	2			2
P. R.				
Partial failure			1	1
Total failure	1	1	1	3
Total	3	1	2	6

June 1969

C. Tolerance

Among the side effects observed in patients treated with L-asparaginase, fever and urticaria must be noted. Reversible shocks were observed in 4 patients; in 3 patients these shocks were preceded by positive skin tests and may thus be due to immunization.

In most patients biological symptoms of slight, moderate or severe toxicity were noted, shown in Table 4; decreases in cholesterol, albumin and fibrin values were the most frequent and early symptoms. Two patients died from hepatic failure with severe fibrinopenia, fall of coagulation factors, increase of bilirubinemia: one of these patients was in hematological remission.

Table 4. *Abnormalities in hepatic tests of patients treated with L-asparaginase*

Cholesterol g/l	≧ 1,50 13 (28%)	1,50—1 25 (53%)	1—0,80 6 (13%)	≦ 0,80 3 (6%)
Indirect bilirubin mg/l	≦ 5 25 (53%)	5—10 14 (30%)	10—20 7 (15%)	20—50 1 (2%)
Transaminases S.G.P.T. (U. Wroblewski)	≦50 30 (64%)	50—100 14 (30%)	100—200 1 (2%)	200—500 2 (4%)
Alkaline phosphatases (U. King)	≦10 23 (50%)	10—20 10 (21%)	20—30 9 (20%)	30—50 5 (9%)
Albuminemia g/l	≧35 19 (40%)	35—25 8 (17%)	25—20 12 (26%)	≦20 8 (17%)

The main interest of L-asparaginase lies in the possibility of combining it with other active drugs.

Professor Jean Bernard in his presentation has already pointed out the interest of a combination including vincristine, daunomycin, prednisone and L-asparaginase in advanced A. L. L. He mentioned also the encouraging preliminary results observed with daunomycin, methotrexate and L-asparaginase in A. M. L. These studies are still in progress.

C. Dioxopiperazine Propane

Further Clinical Experiences with ICRF 159

K. Hellmann

Imperial Cancer Research Fund, London, W. C. 2

Since the preliminary clinical assessment of ICRF 159 in acute leukemia [1] in which results on nine. patients were reviewed, a further four patients with acute monocytic and three with acute lymphocytic leukaemia have been studied. There has also been one additional patient with lymphosarcoma.

In all these cases the same pattern of activity as with the first series of patients has been repeated. At a dose level of 20—30 mg/kg over a period of four days at a time a sharp leukopenic effect is evident, though platelets are much less if at all affceted. The haemoglobin levels generally remained unchanged.

The decline in cell count was in every case steeper for the immature leukaemic cells than for normal leukocytic cells. It was not possible however to achieve a complete clearance of leukaemic cells from the peripheral blood and the bone marrow appearance remained essentially unchanged in all these patients.

The leukopenic effect was independent of any previous treatment and as in the first series of cases no cross-resistance with any of the currently used anti-leukaemic drugs including asparaginase and cytosine arabinoside was observed.

Again as in the first series of cases the drug was very well tolerated with no evidence of gastro-intestinal disturbances. Thinning of the scalp hair was probably increased in most and definitely in some patients. Clinically nearly all patients mentioned that they felt much better.

The main problem therefore in using ICRF 159 as an anti-leukaemic and possibly also as an anticancer agent generally lies in increasing the degree of selectivity against cancer cells.

This may be a problem of administration. At present the drug is given for a maximum of four days, but other dosage schedules might be more effective. Much seems to depend on the individual sensitivities of the cells and when in their life cycle the drug is presented to them.

In recent experiments in which the effect of ICRF 159 on the spontaneous metastases of the mouse Lewis lung tumour was examined it was observed that although the drug (at 30 mg/kg) did not affect the growth of the primary tumour, it totally inhibited the appearance of lung metastases. One possible explanation of this effect is that the secondary tumour cells may be more sensitive to the drug than the primary tumour cells, but clearly other explanations are possible, particularly that ICRF 159 may prevent implantation of metastases. Indeed it is this aspect of its activity that may be more important than the non-selective destruction of leukaemic cells.

Reference

1. Hellmann, K., Newton, K. A., Whitmore, D. N., Hanham, I., Bond, J. V.: Preliminary clinical assessment of ICRF 159 in acute leukaemia and lymphosarcoma. Brit. med. J. **1**, 822 (1969).

Preliminary Data on Acute Leukemia Treatment with ICRF 159

G. Mathé, J. L. Amiel, M. Hayat, F. de Vassal, L. Schwarzenberg, M. Schneider, C. Jasmin, and C. Rosenfeld

Institut Cancérologique et d'Immunogénétique, Hôpital Paul Brousse 14, avenue Paul-Vaillant Couturier, et Service d'Hématologie Institut Gustave Roussy 16 bis, avenue Paul-Vaillant Couturier, 94 — Villejuif

With 3 Figures

We have treated 10 patients with acute leukaemia, 7 lymphoblastic and 3 myeloblastic, with ICRF 159 or dioxopiperazine propane (Fig. 1). All these patients were resistant to all the drugs so far available. The daily doses were 300 mg/m².

```
   O                          O
    \\                       //
     C-CH2           CH2-C
HN<         >N-CH2-CH-N<        >NH
     C-CH2           |     CH-C
    //               R         \\
   O                             O
```

Fig. 1. ICRF 159: [(±-1,2-bis (3,5-dioxopiperazin-1-yl) propane]

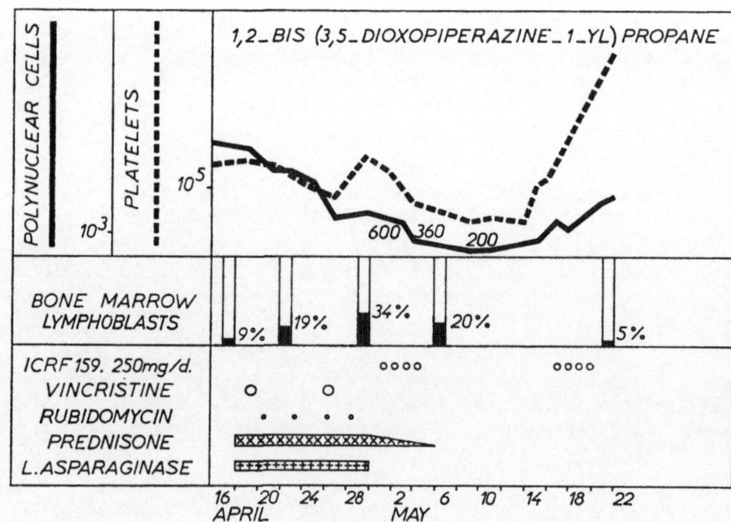

Fig. 2. Complete remission induce by ICRF 159 in a patient resistant to the combination of vincristine, rubidomycin, prednisone and L-asparaginase

We have obtained 2 complete remissions, in lymphoblastic leukaemia cases: they are shown in Fig. 2 and 3.

In other cases, specially with myeloblastic leukaemia, the number of leukaemic cells fell temporarily, but they increased again under treatment. No toxicity was observed, with the exception of the appearance of peripheral-cytopenia.

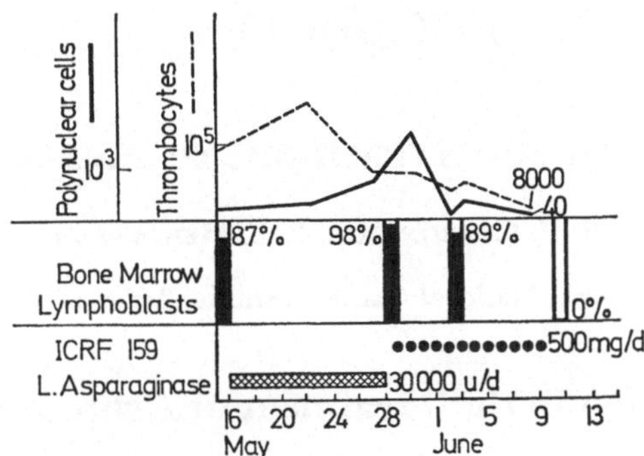

Fig. 3. Complete remission induce by ICRF 159 in a patient resistant to L-asparaginase

The selection of patients undergoing treatment with this drug, that are patients resistant to all previously available treatments is an unfavourable selection; this gives hope that it could induce remissions with a higher frequency on patients in the early phases of the disease.

Reference

Hellmann, K., Newton, K. A., Whitmore, D. N., Hanham, I., Bond, J. V.: Preliminary clinical assessment of ICRF 159 in acute leukaemia and lymphosarcoma. Brit. med. J. 1, 822 (1969).

D. Other Drugs

New Drugs in the Treatment of Acute Leukemia

P. P. CARBONE and E. S. HENDERSON

The Medicine Branch, National Cancer Institute, Bethesda, Maryland 20014

New Drugs in the Treatment of Acute Leukemia

In this brief review the term "new drugs" will be used in the broad sense of drug activities not previously appreciated or fully exploited. This will permit discussion not only of chemical entities not previously available, but agents whose potential for arresting leukemic cell growth has not been adequately defined. Drugs of the latter category include asparaginase and daunorubicin, currently undergoing extensive clinical study, but which, as subjects of earlier discussion at this symposium, are excluded from this report. Included (Table 1) are drugs such as bis-β-chloroethyl

Table 1. *New drugs for acute leukemia*

I. Previously untested
   - Poly-I-C
   - CCNU
   - Pseudourea

II. Currently undergoing initial trials in man
   - ICBM
   - Camptothecin
   - Epipodophyllotoxin
   - Dibromo dulcitol

III. Previously used with inconclusive results in man
   - Actinomycin D
   - 5-Fluorouracil
   - BCNU
   - Vinblastine

nitrosourea (BCNU), vinblastine (VLB), actinomycin D, and 5-fluorouracyl, which have been used to inconclusive advantage in the past; dibromo dulcitol (DBD), imidazole carboximide bis-β-chlorethyl (ICBM), and camptothecin which have received only preliminary evaluation. The animal screening and toxicity data for a selected group of clinically new and untried entities, chloro-cyclohexyl nitrosourea (CCNU), polyinosinic/polycytidylic (Poly-IC), demethyl-epipodophyllotoxin-thenylidine-glycoside (PTG), and pseudourea, will also be reviewed.

New Chemical Structures

The new and untested chemicals have been identified for study using the screening system of the Cancer Chemotherapy National Service Center. Because of the utility of murine leukemia L 1210 as a predictor of anti-leukemic activity in man [10], this test system serves as the primary screening for candidate agents. CCNU, pseudourea, camptothecin, ICBM, DBD and PTG were all positive with this assay.

Polyinosinic-polycytidoylic acid (Poly IC)

(NSC 120949) is a synthetic, double-stranded RNA polymer originally described by Field and coworkers to cause interferon production *in vitro* [9]. Poly IC also causes enhanced rejection of skin grafts and inhibition of animal tumors including L 1210 [1, 17]. There is no apparent schedule dependency with use of Poly IC.

Toxicity of Poly IC in monkeys and dogs is mainly a result of its ability to effect intravascular coagulation [10 a, 13]. Doses of 0.3 mg/kg or less are tolerated in both species with reversible changes in the coagulation factors and liver enzymes. No clinical studies have been done as yet but studies of clinical toxicology and interferon induction are comtemplated. The interferon induction and immune enhancement would have obvious clinical usefulness for studies in patients with acute leukemia.

CCNU

CCNU (Table 2) is a member of the substituted nitrosoureas synthesized by Montgomery and co-workers [15]. Like BCNU it exhibits striking activity against L 1210 leukemia, a single optimum dose resulting in cures of the early disease. Schabel et al. have further demonstrated therapeutic synergism [22] between this compound and cytarabine in the same tumor. CCNU alkylates, but may well have additional activity as an antimetabolite [21]. It is highly lipid soluble and thus is readily absorbed from the gastrointestinal tract and widely distributed throughout the body. It is rapidly degrated to cyclohexylamine, dicyclohexylurea and several undefined metabolites, the plasma $T^1/_2$ for the native compound being less than

Table 2. *Cyclohexyl-chloroethyl nitrosourea (CCNU) (NSC No. 79037)*

Animal tumor activity:	L1210: ILS > 650% single i. p.
Animal toxicity:	mouse: LD_{10} 150 (i. p.) 290 mg/m² (p. o.) dog: MTD 3.0 mg/m²/d X 15 monkey: MTD 8.0 mg/m²/d X 15
Limiting toxicity:	myelosuppression, dose related hepatotoxicity
Dose form:	oral: capsules of 20 and 440 mg i. v.: not available
Human toxicity:	single dose: MTD: ~ 130 mg/m² divided dose (one day): ~ 100 mg/m² signs and symptoms: nausea, vomiting, pancytopenia (reversible)

10 min [20]. CCNU was chosen for clinical trial because of its similarity to BCNU on the one hand, and the relatively lower incidence in delayed toxicity in animal studies on the other. To date its toxicity in man appears similar qualitatively to BCNU but with a lower maximum tolerated dose (130 mg/m^2 vs. 300 mg/m^2 as a single dose). Whether or not therapeutic effects will be altered by this difference remains to be determined.

Pseudourea

Pseudourea (Table 3) is an anthracine derivative with significant activity against L 1210. It is most active in mice given in multiple doses on a single day, resulting in a median increased life span of 200 per cent, and in cures in a minority of mice so treated. Toxicity is primarily bone marrow directed, but hepatic and renal toxicity have been observed in dogs and monkeys. There is a suggestion that in Rhesus monkeys the drug may selectively spare megakaryocytes. The compound's major drawback is its extremely curtailed water solubility, coupled with negligible gastrointestinal absorption. No clinical trials have been initiated with this drug [4].

Table 3. *Pseudourea (NSC 56054)*

Animal tumor activity:	L1210: ILS > 200 q 6 h d 1 3/10 cures q 3 h d 1
Animal toxicity:	mouse: LD_{50} ~ 450 mg/m^2/d X 1
	dog: ~ 50 mg/m^2/d X 28 I.V.
	monkey: ~ 35 mg/m^2/d X 28
	myelotoxic, hepatotoxic, and nephrotoxic
	megakaryocytes spared in rhesus monkeys
Dose formulation:	sterile solution 30 mg/10 ml
	propylene glycol stored at −10° C
	dilute in aqueous vehicle other than saline
Solubility is a problem; drug is not absorbed orally; no clinical trials to date	

Imidazole-carboxamide-bis-β-chloroethyl Triazino

This compound (Table 4) is a congener of imidazole-carboxamide dimethyltriazino (NSC 45 388) a drug which has shown activity against melanosarcoma. Like other members of its class it appears to act both as an inhibitor of purine synthesis and as an alkylating agent. It has a broad spectrum of antitumor activity in animals including outstanding effectiveness in the L 1210 assay system. In this tumor, single or widely spaced dosing is clearly superior. Myelotoxicity is the primary adverse side effect in animals, whereas the limiting clinical toxicity has been gastrointestinal e. g. severe nausea and vomiting. Hepatic damage was observed in dogs and monkeys, and in previously treated patients with acute leukemia. The drug is poorly soluble in aqueous solution, and for this reason it has been given orally in the limited clinical trials to date. Absorption by this route has been quite variable [7 a], GI toxicity has been severe and dose limiting, and results in the few acute leukemic patients treated thus far have been disappointing. A parenteral dosage form has been developed and clinical trials with this formulation are imminent.

Table 4. *Imidazole-carboxamide-bis-chloroethyl-triazeno (ICBM) (NSC 82196)*

Animal tumor activity:	L1210: ILS = 250 q 3—7 d i. p. cures with single large dose S 180, CA 755, W 256 } active
Animal toxicity:	mouse: LD_{50} 4.0—6.0 g/m² p. o. dog: MTD 100 mg/m²/day monkey: MTD < 250 mg/m²/day bone marrow, liver—often delayed
Dose form:	30 mg capsules (stored frozen in dark) parenteral dosage form now available
Human toxicology:	poor and erratic absorption MTD ≤ 1000 mg/m²/week or 500 mg/m²/day X 5 Gastrointestinal (nausea, vomiting, diarrhea) limiting. Hepatotoxicity seen in previously treated acute leukemics

Dibromodulcitol (DBD)

DBD (Table 5) has had considerable clinical exposure in lymphomas and chronic leukemia [8]. Unlike the closely related dibromomannitol it is active against leukemia L 1210 and will accordingly soon be evaluated in acute leukemia patients. Toxicity in both animals and man is chiefly that of bone marrow injury. SELAWRY and co-workers at the Veterans Administration Hospital of Washington are currently conducting human toxicology studies which thus far demonstrate severe and prolonged pancytopenias at dosages over 100 mg/m²/day p.o. The drug is well absorbed orally, is metabolized, and excreted in the urine. The plasma $T^1/_2$ is approximately six hours [3, 14].

Table 5. *Dibromodulcitol (DBD) (NSC 104800)*

Animal tumor activity:	L1210: ILS: 55% i. p. q 2.4 d W256: TWI: 97% i. p. qd P388: inactive
Animal toxicity:	mouse: LD_{50} 1,500 mg/m²/day X 1 dog: MTD 100 mg/m²/day X 15 monkey: 60 mg/m²/day X 15 bone marrow, liver and gastrointestinal toxicity
Dosage form:	oral: 25 mg tablets
Animal pharmacology:	metabolized excreted in urine plasma $T^1/_2$ ~ 6 hours
Human toxicity:	daily p. o. schedule: MTD ~ 100 mg/m²/day delayed, prolonged pancytopenia

4′-Demethyl-epipodophyllotoxin-thenylidene-glycoside (PTG)

PTG (Table 6) is a podophyllotoxin derivative which, unlike other podophyllotoxin derivatives, exhibits effectiveness against both systemic and intracranially innoculated leukemia L 1210. It further lacks cardiovascular toxicity of the severity

Table 6. *4'-Demethyl-epipodophyllotoxin-thenylidene-glycoside (PTG) (NSC 122810) (VM 26 — Sandoz)*

Animal tumor activity:	L1210: ILS 286% 2X/week CNS-L 1210 ILS 150% also active VS. W256, P1534, P815, Ehrlichs
Animal toxicity:	mouse: LD_{50} 48 mg/m² single dose monkey: MTD 14 mg/m²/day X 14
Major toxicities:	myelosuppression; reversible hypotension
Pharmacology:	excreted in urine and bile ? metabolism plasma $T^1/_2$ (rats) ~ 34 min.
Dosage form:	5 and 25 mg ampules for i. v. injection
Clinical trials:	just initiated

exhibited by other members of its class. PTG's major toxicity is myelosuppression, reversible hypotension occurring in animals only after larger doses. The LD_{50} in the mouse is 48 mg/m² following a single I.V. dose. In the monkey the maximum tolerated dose on a daily I.V. schedule is 14 mg/m²/day. The drug is excreted in bile and urine; the plasma $T^1/_2$ being 34 minutes in mice, and longer in larger animals. PTG is currently undergoing initial clinical trials in the chemotherapy unit of the Washinton, D. C. Veterans Administration Hospital under the direction of Dr. OLEG SELAWRY.

Camptothecin

Camptothecin lactone (NCS-94000; Table 7) is an alkyloid of *Camptotheca acuminata Nyssaceae* with activity against both L 1210 and the Walker carcinosarcoma. Its primary toxicity is gastrointestinal ulceration, to a degree which pre-

Table 7. *Camptothecin (NSC 94600)*

Animal tumor activity:	L1210: ILS 102% p 7 d W256: active	
Animal toxicity:	mouse, LD_{50} i. p.	♂ 211 mg/m² ♀ 126 mg/m²
	LD_{50} p. o.	80 mg/m²
	dog (beagle), MTD	3 mg/m²/day X 14 80 mg/m²/week X 6
	monkey,	15 mg/m²/daily X 14
Major toxicity:	gastrointestional ulceration, emesis, hepatitis, nephritis, bone marrow depression. Intermittent parenteral doses best tolerated	
Dosage formulation:	camptothecin, lactone, sodium salt, 5 mg vial, reconstituted with water extreme shortage of drug	
Human studies:	no data to date	

cludes oral administration. Activity is greatest, and toxicity least, when the compound is administered intravenously by an intermittent dosage schedule [18]. In mice the drug is rapidly cleared from the plasma ($T^{1}/_{2}$ 27 min) and localized primarily in the gastrointestinal tract, liver and kidneys. It is largely metabolized to as yet undefined end product [11]. The major limitation to its use is the extreme shortage of the compound. It has been started in the clinic on a restricted basis at the National Cancer Institute's Baltimore Chemotherapy Unit for pharmacological and toxicological evaluation.

Old Drugs

In the feverish search for new drugs it is appropriate to consider whether or not existing agents have been overlooked or ignored because of inadequate preliminary studies. The standard method for evaluating anti-leukemic compounds is in trials of remission induction. Unless significant effects are seen in drug is often discarded, frequently despite many inadequate trials and usually after the evaluation of only one or two arbitrary dose schedules. Table 8 lists several examples of drugs whose

Table 8. *Clinical trials in leukemia suggesting anti-tumor activity of rarely used drugs*

Induction	*Maintenance*	*%CR*	*Duration of remission* [a]	*Reference*
VCR+P	MTX-6MP-CYT	—		Holland, 1966
	MTX-6MP-CYT-*BCNU*	—		
VCR+P	*VCR*		11 months	Colebatch, 1969
	6MP ⇄ MTX	—	406 days	Leikin et al., 1969
	6MP+*ACT*-D ⇄ MTX+*HN2*	—	720 days	
VCR 0.015—0.02 mg/kg/week; *VLB* 0.15—0.2 mg/kg/week		45% [b]		Massimo, 1969

[a] Includes complete plus partial remissions.
[b] Most reported to be resistent to VCR.

activities have been discounted at one or another phase of therapy. BCNU, given daily as an induction agent, resulted in severe and often fatal toxicity, and was abandoned. When added to an effective remission maintenance protocol, superior remission durations were observed [12]. Its optimum dose and schedule and ultimate assessment as an anti-leukemic therapy have not been established. Vincristine was clearly shown to be ineffective as maintenance in previously treated patients with acute lymphoblastic leukemia. This judgement has been recently questioned by the report of the Australian Cooperative Group [7] which successfully employed VCR alone during remission and by the improved results reported by the Acute Leukemia Group B when VCR was added to 6-MP or MTX maintenance programs [6]. Similarly the intermittent administration of actinomycin D and nitrogen mustard to 6-MP-MTX maintenance has resulted in longer leukemic control [16], and the addition of vinca-leukoblastin to vincristine has been reported to be effective remission induction therapy for patients resistant to vincristine alone [19]. While all of these observations require additional confirmation, they collectively caution us not to be too hasty in discarding such candidate agents, particularly those which have shown unquestioned activity against non-leukemic neoplasms, but rather to carefully reconsider their use in the light of the increasing knowledge of the growth kinetics and biochemical nature of leukemic cell lines.

Summary

Preclinical evaluation of several new drugs slated for clinical trial in human malignancy have recently been completed by the chemotherapy division of the National Cancer Institute. These drugs include a nitrosourea (CCNU), imidazole-carboxamide-bis-B-chloroethyl triazino, dibromodulcitol, pseudourea, a podophyllotoxin derivative, a plant alkyloid camptothecin lactone, and a synthetic polyriboside (poly IC). The animal tumor responses, pharmacology, and toxicology of these agents are discussed.

References

1. Adamson, R.: Personal Communication.
2. Carter, S. K., Newman, J. W.: Nitrosoureas: 1,3-Bis(2-chloroethyl-1-nitrosourea (NSC-409962; BCNU) and 1,-(2-chloroethyl)-3-cyclohexyl-1-nitrosourea (NSC-79037; CCNU). Clinical Brochure. Cancer Chemother. Rep. **1**, 115—152 (1968).
3. Carter, S. K.: Dibromoducitol (NSC-104800). Clinical Brochure. Cancer Chemother. Rep. **1**, 165—178 (1968).
4. — 2,2′-(9,10-Anthrylenedinethylene)-bis-[2-thiopseudourea], dihydrochloride, dihydrate (NSC-56054). Clinical Brochure. Cancer Chemother. Rep. **1**, 153—177 (1968).
5. — Newman, J. W.: 5(or 4)-[3,3-Bis(2-chloroethyl)-1-triazeno]-imidazole-4(or 5)-carboxamide (NSC-82196). Clinical Brochure. Cancer Chemother. Rep. **1**, 63—80 (1968).
6. Chevalier, L., Glidewell, O.: Schedule of 6-mercaptopurine and effect of inducer dose in prolongation of remission maintenance in acute leukemia. Proc. Amer. Ass. Cancer Lancet **1968 II**, 869.
7. Colebatch, J. H., Baikie, A. G., Clark, A. C. L., Jones, D. L., Lee, C. W. G., Lewis, T. C., Newman, N. M.: Cyclic regimen for childhood leukemia. Letter to the Editor. Lancet **2**, 869 (1968).

7 a. De Vita, V. T.: Personal Communication.

8. Eckhardt, S.: Chronic myelogenous leukemia and its treatment with dibromomannitol. Proc. Vth International Congress of Chemotherapy. **3**, 259—264 (1967).
9. Field, H. K., Titell, A. A., Lampson, G. P., Hillman, M. R.: Inducers of interferon and host resistance. IV Double-stranded, replicative form RNA (NS2-FF-RNA) from E. coli infected with MS-2 coliphage. Proc. nat. Acad. Sci. (Wash.) **58**, 2102—2108 (1967).
10. Goldin, A., Serpick, A. A., Mantel, N.: Experimental screening procedures and clinical predictability value. A commentary. Cancer Chemother. Rep. **50**, 173—218 (1966).

10 a. Gralnick, H., Henry, P.: Personal Communication.

11. Guarino, A. M., Hart, L. G., Call, J. B., Oliverio, V. T.: Studies of the physiological disposition of the antitumor agent, camptothecin sodium (NSC 100880) in rodents. Proc. Amer. Ass. Cancer Res. 10, 33 (1969).
12. Holland, J. F.: Progress in the treatment of acute leukemia. In: Perspectives in Leukemia. New York: Grune & Stratton 1968, p. 217.
13. Homan, E. R., Zendzian, R. R., Adamson, R. H.: Some aspects of the pharmacology and toxicology of polyinosinic acid. Proc. Amer. Ass. Cancer Res. **10**, 40 (1969).
14. Institoris, L., Horvath, I. P., Pethes, G.: Some characteristic features of the biotransport of the cytostatic agent 1,6-dibromo-1,6-dideoxy-dulcitol. Int. J. Cancer **2**, 21—25 (1967).
15. Johnston, T. P., McCaleb, G. S., Opliger, P. S., Montgomery, J. A.: The synthesis of potential anticancer agent. XXXVI. N-nitrosoureas. II. Haloalkyl derivatives. J. med. Chem. **9**, 892—911 (1966).

16. Leiken, S., Brubaker, C., Hartmann, J., Murphy, M. L., Wolff, J.: The use of combination therapy in leukemia remission. Cancer **22**, 427—432 (1969).
17. Levy, H. B., Law, L. W., Rabson, A. S.: The effect of polyinosinic-cytidylic acid on tumor growth. Proc. Amer. Ass. Cancer Res. **10**, 49 (1969).
18. Livingston, R. B., Carter, S. K.: Camptothecin, sodium salt (NSC100,880). Clinical brochure. NCI.
19. Massimo, L., Mori, P. G., Cottafava, F., Fossati-Guglielmoni, A.: Vincristine plus vinblastine in acute childhood leukemia. Lancet **15**, 469 (1969).
20. Oliverio, V. T., Vietzke, W. M., Williams, M. K., Adamson, R. H.: Pharmacological studies of the carcinostatic 1-(2-chloroethyl)-3-cyclohexyl-1-nitrosourea (CCNU) in animals. Proc. Amer. Ass. Cancer Res. **9**, 56 (1968).
21. Pettillo, R. F., Narkates, A. T., Burns, J.: Microbiological evaluation of BCNU. Cancer Res. **24**, 1222—1228 (1964).
22. Schabel, F. M., Jr.: In vivo leukemic cell kill kinetics and "Curability" in experimental system. In: The University of Texas M. D. Anderson Hospital and Tumor Institute. The Proliferation and Spread of Neoplastic Cells. Baltimore: Williams and Wilkins 1968, pp. 379—408.
23. Selawry, O. S., Hansen, H. H.: Initial clinical trial with chloroethylcyclohexylnitrosourea (CCNU, NSC-79037). Proc. Amer. Ass. Cancer Res. **10**, 78 (1969).

E. Immunotherapy

Active Immunotherapy of L 1210 Leukemia Applied After the Graft of Tumor Cells[1]

G. Mathé and P. Pouillart

With the technical assistance of Françoise Lapeyraque, Institut de Cancérologie et d'Immunogénétique, Hôpital Paul-Brousse, 14, Avenue Paul-Vaillant-Couturier, 94-Villejuif, France

With 7 Figures

Various authors have demonstrated that the growth of a tumour can be retarded by pre-treatment of the host *before* grafting the tumour, by either irradiated tumour cells [1] or by the adjuvants of immunity, BCG [2—5] and Corynebacterium parvum [6—8]. In these instances, the therapy has begun before the onset of growth of the tumour.

In the present state of our knowledge of the antigens of human tumour cells, one cannot envisage the application of the immunotherapy of cancer in a preventive form, that is, before the onset of the disease. On the other hand, one can see the possibility of applying the technique in a curative role. It is for this reason that we wish to know if it is able to be effective when it is applied *after* the development of the neoplasm, that is, when the animal is already carrying the tumour cell antigens. We have already shown that this is a possibility [9] and described some of the conditions under which it was effective.

We are now making a detailed study of these conditions by a series of experiments carried out on transplantable leukaemia, on a virus-induced leukaemia and on spontaneous leukaemia. The present paper is concerned with the results of experiments on a transplantable leukaemia.

Materials and Methods

1. The Leukaemia

We have chosen the L 1210 leukaemia maintained in DBA/2 mice, as a graftable leukaemia. This was transplanted into (C57Bl/6×DBA/2)F1 mice aged three months.

[1] This work was supported by a grant from I.N.S.E.R.M., No. 66—235.

2. First Experiment

A comparison of the effect upon leukaemia produced by the injection of 10^4 cells, of a single or repeated injections of various adjuvants, and irradiated leukaemic cells given after the graft of the leukaemia.

Two hundred and eighteen mice received 10^4 L 1210 leukaemic tumour cells, by subcutaneous injection; they were then divided at random into 10 groups of 20 animals and one group of 18. The first group acted as controls. Groups 2 and 3 were treated with living BCG[2]: group 2, by a single intravenous injection of 1 mg 24 hours after the graft; group 3, by 5 injections of 1 mg every fourth day, beginning 24 hours after the graft. Groups 4 and 5 were treated by Bordetella pertussis[2]: 1 mg intraperitoneally as a single injection (group 4), or repeated 5 times at 4 days intervals (group 5). Groups 6 and 7 were treated by Corynebacterium parvum[2]: 1 mg intraperitoneally, either as a single injection (group 6), or repeated 5 times at 4 day intervals (group 7). Groups 8 and 9 were treated by Mycobacterium cheiloni[3]: 1 mg intraperitoneally as a single dose (group 8), or repeated 5 times at 4 day intervals (group 9). Groups 10 and 11 were treated by injection(s) of 10^7 L 1210 leukaemic cells that had been irradiated with 15,000 rads, either as a single injection (group 10), or repeated five times at 4 day intervals (group 11); the conditions of the irradiation in vitro were as follows: a suspension of cells was prepared containing 5×10^7 cells per mm^3; the suspension was divided into 4.5 ml aliquots and put into Petri dishes, irradiated at 250 Kv, 12 mA (0.2 copper filtration), at a dose rate of 325 r/min, the source being 130 cm from the dishes.

The cumulative survival of the animals in the different groups were studied and comparisons made between them.

3. Second Experiment

The comparison of the effect of active immunotherapy by BCG, or irradiated leukaemic cells or by the association of these two methods, given after grafting the leukaemia, as opposed to the effect of active immunotherapy applied before the graft.

a) Administration of Immunotherapy 14 Days Before the Graft of the Leukaemia

Thirty-seven (C57Bl/6×DBA/2) F1 mice were given 10^4 L 1210 leukaemic cells subcutaneously. Fourteen days previously, they had been divided, at random, into 4 groups: the first (11 animals) acted as controls and were not treated; the second (10 animals) had been given 1 mg of BCG intravenously, which was then repeated every fourth day, beginning on the fourteenth day before the graft. The third group (6 animals) had been treated on the fourteenth day before the graft by a single subcutaneous injection of 10^7 leukaemic cells that had been irradiated with 15,000 rads, as described above. The fourth group (10 animals) has been given a combination of both these treatments.

The tumour volume was measured every second day and the date of death was recorded and a cumulative survival curve constructed for these animals.

[2] From the Institut Pasteur, Paris, France.
[3] From the Laboratoire Joly, 95-Eaubonne, France.

b) The Administration of Immunotherapy, 24 Hours, 4 Days or 6 Days, After the Graft of the Leukaemia

These experiments only differed from the preceding ones by the dates of injection of the irradiated leukaemic cells or the first injection of BCG being made on the 24th hour, or the fourth or sixth day before the graft of the leukaemia.

In the first sub-group, receiving immunotherapy 24 hours after the graft of the leukaemia, 10 animals received BCG alone, 9 received irradiated leukaemic cells, and 9 a combination of these two treatments. In a second sub-group, who were given immunotherapy 4 days after the graft of the leukaemia, 8 animals received BCG alone, 9 irradiated cells, and 9 a combination of these two treatments. In a third sub-group, who received immunotherapy on the 6th day after the graft, 11 animals received BCG alone, 9 irradiated cells and 9 a combination of these two treatments.

4. Third Experiment

Effect of active immunotherapy applied after the graft of the leukaemia, accordind to the number of leukaemic cells that were grafted.

Five hundred and twenty-three (C57Bl/6×DBA/2) F1 female mice were used for this experiment. They were divided into 6 groups at random and were injected subcutaneously with a variable number of L 1210 leukaemic cells, according to the different groups: 88 mice in group I received 10^7 cells; 90 mice in group II received 10^6; 90 mice in group III received 10^5; 84 mice in group IV received 10^4; 86 mice in group V received 10^3 and 85 mice in group VI received 10^2 leukaemic cells.

The animals in each of these groups were then subdivided into 4 groups, A, B, C and D. The animals in group A acted as controls. The animals in group B received, during the 24 hours which followed the graft of the L 1210 leukaemia, an intravenous injection of 1 mg of BCG; this injection was repeated every fourth day for 30 days. The animals in group C received, during the first 24 hours which followed the tumour graft, a single injection of 10^7 L 1210 leukaemic cells subcutaneously, which had previously been irradiated in vitro with a dose of 15,000 rads as described above. The mice in group D were treated by both the BCG and the irradiated leukaemic cells.

Results

1. First Experiment

Comparison of the effect, on leukaemia produced by the injection of 10^4 cells, of a single or repeated injection of various adjuvants, or irradiated leukaemic cells given after the graft of the leukaemia.

It can be seen, in Fig. 1, that among the adjuvants or substances used for their possible adjuvant properties, only BCG, when it was given repeatedly, was able to give any appreciable result. This treatment enabled a certain number of the animals to be cured. On the fortieth day of the experiment, the difference in mortality between the animals treated with BCG and the controls was significant ($p < 1$ per cent).

It can be seen also that the mortality of the mice can be increased by the ad-

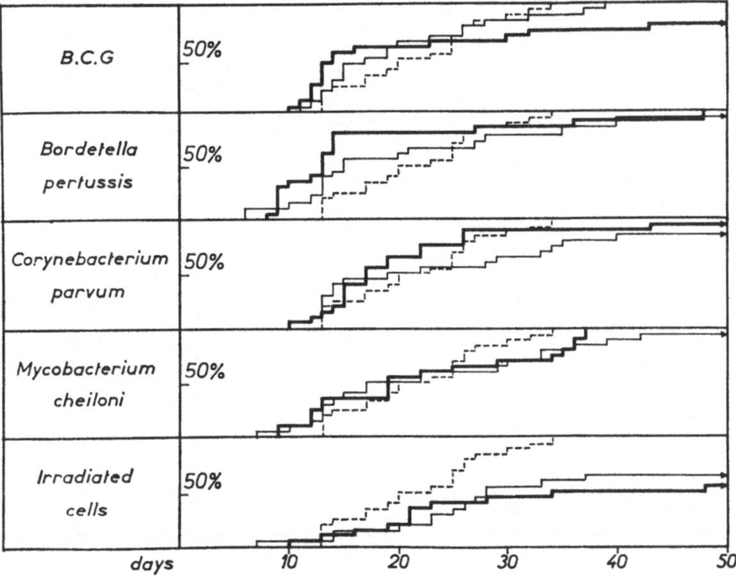

—— Controls; —— 1 injection 24 h after tumor graft; ------- 5 injections one each 4th day

Fig. 1. Cumulative survival of mice carrying L 1210 leukaemia, not treated or treated by adjuvants (one injection or several injections) or irradiated leukaemic cells (one injection or several injections)

ministration of certain adjuvants, particularly Bordetella pertussis. This seems to be mainly due to toxicity rather than immunological enhancement for, in none of the experiments was the tumour volume of the animals treated with the adjuvant greater than that in the control animals. This slight increase of early mortality is also seen in these experiments after the repeated injections of BCG. This effect on the early deaths was not present in all the experiments, as will be shown later.

In Fig. 1, it can be seen that the effect of irradiated leukaemic cells is better than that of BCG, which was the best of the adjuvants tried in this experiment, and repeated injections of the irradiated leukaemic cells were not notably different from the effect of a single injection.

2. Second Experiment

The effect of active immunotherapy from BCG, or irradiated leukaemic cells or a combination of these two, applied after giving the leukaemic graft, as compared to the effects of active immunotherapy applied before the graft.

This experiment, made as in the preceding one, upon 10^4 grafted leukaemic cells, shows first the difference of action according to the date of giving the BCG and the irradiated leukaemic cells. The BCG was very active when it was given 14 days before the tumour graft (the difference between the controls is very significant: $p < 0.1$), whilst the leukaemic cells had hardly any effect (no effect upon the tumour volume and a non-significant prolongation of the survival) (Fig. 2).

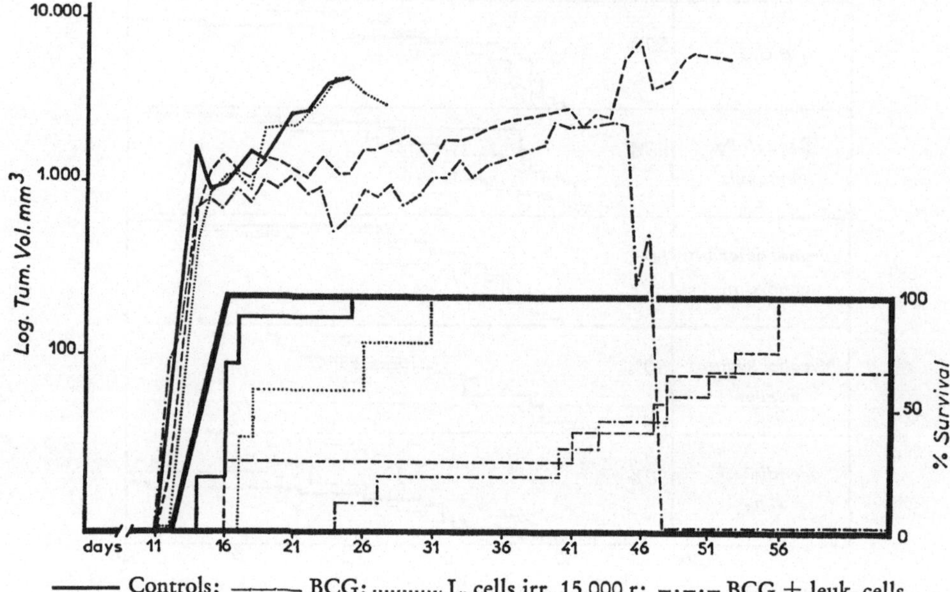

——— Controls; ——— BCG; .... L. cells irr. 15,000 r; —·—·— BCG + leuk. cells

Fig. 2. Tumor volume and cumulative survival of mice grafted with L 1210 leukaemia and not treated, or treated by BCG (first injection 14 days before the graft and injections repeated every fourth days) or irradiated leukaemic cells (one injection 14 days before the graft), or association of both

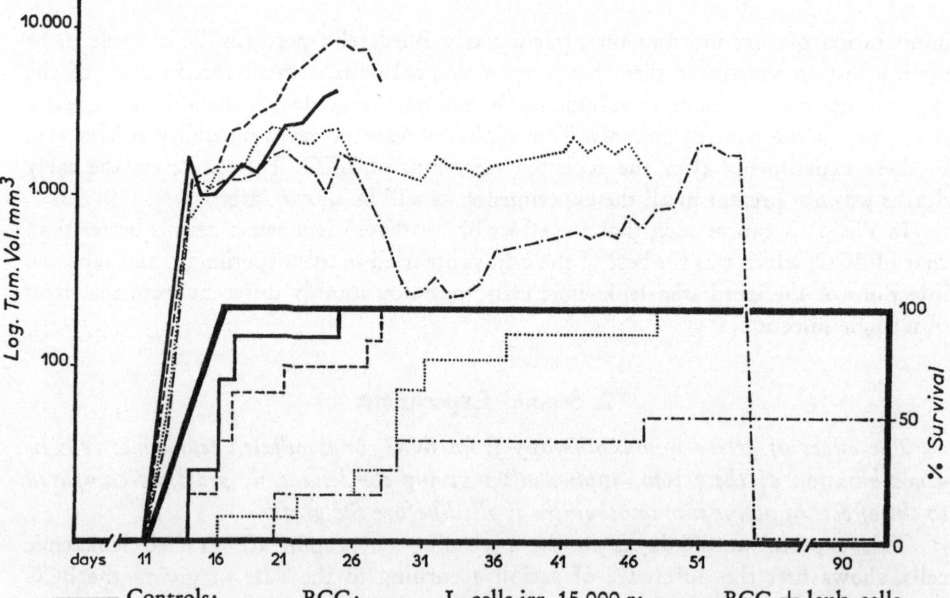

——— Controls; ——— BCG; .... L. cells irr. 15,000 r; —·—·— BCG + leuk. cells

Fig. 3. Tumor volume and cumulative survival of mice grafted with L 1210 leukaemia and not treated or treated by BCG (first injection 24 hours after the graft and injections repeated each four days), or irradiated leukaemic cells (one injecttion 24 hours after the graft), or association of both

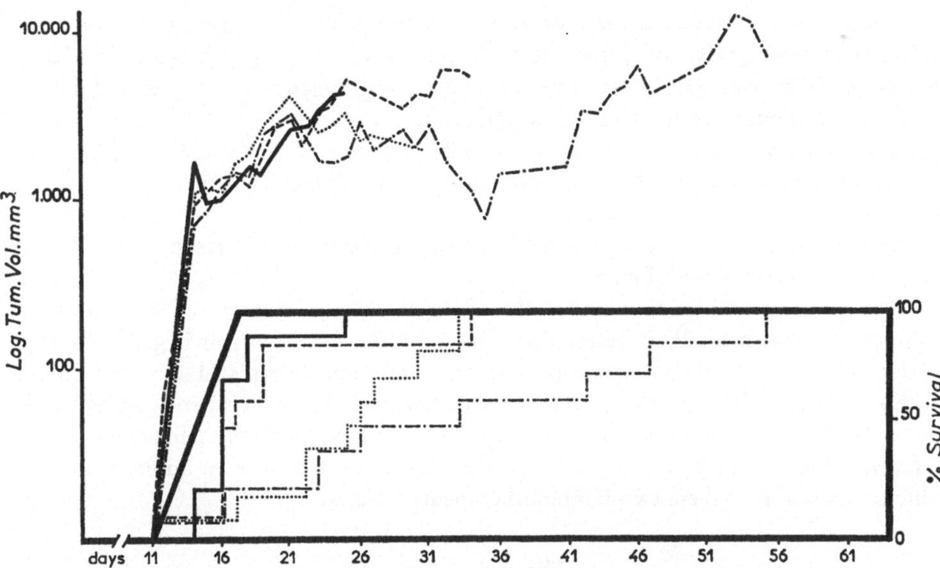

Fig. 4. Tumor volume and cumulative survival of mice grafted with L 1210 leukamia and not treated, or treated by BCG (first injection 4 days after the graft and injections repeated each four days), or irradiated leukaemic cells (one injection 24 hours after the graft), or ciation of both

——— Controls; – – – BCG; · · · · · L. cells irr. 15,000 r; –·–·– BCG + leuk. cells

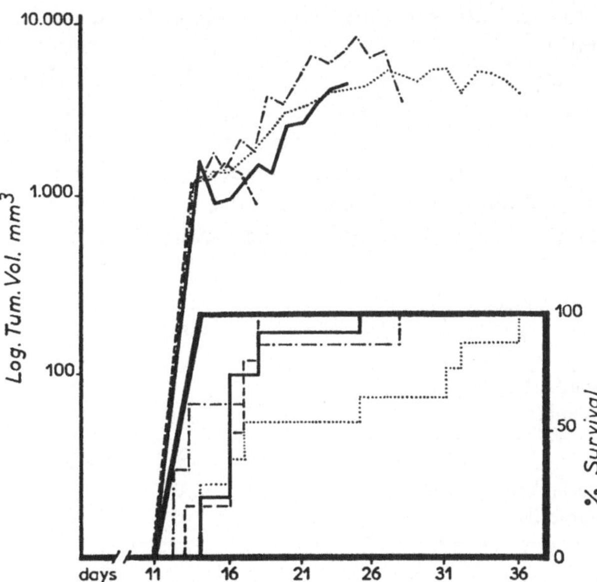

Fig. 5. Tumor volume and cumulative survival of mice grafted with L 1210 leukaemia and not treated, or treated by BCG (first injection 6 days after the graft and injections repeated each four days), or irradiated leukaemic cells (one injection 6 days after the graft), or association of both

——— Controls; – – – BCG; · · · · · L. cells irr. 15,000 r; –·–·– BCG + leuk. cells

The irradiated leukaemic cells were very active when they were given 24 hours after the tumour graft, the difference with the controls is very significant ($p < 0.1$), whilst the BCG was hardly effective (no effect upon the tumour volume and a non-significant prolongation of the survival) (Fig. 3).

The irradiated tumour cells were still effective on the prolongation of the survival when they were given 4 days after the graft of the leukaemia ($p < 5$ per cent) (Fig. 4).

On the sixth day, no effect could be detected either on the mean survival time or on the tumour volume (Fig. 5).

This experiment also shows that the effect of the combination of BCG and the irradiated leukaemic cells is better than that of BCG, even when it is given 14 days before the graft of the leukaemia (a significant difference of $p < 1$ per cent on the 40th day), or to those given by irradiated leukaemic cells, even when they had been given 24 hours after the graft, or 4 days after the graft of the leukaemia (a significant difference of $p < 1$ per cent on the 30th day). There is an addition or possible potentiation of these two immunotherapeutic effects.

3. Third Experiment

The effect of active immunotherapy applied after the graft of the leukaemia, according to the number of tumour cells injected.

Fig. 6 shows the cumulative survival curves of the animals, according to the number of tumour cells with which they were grafted. It will be seen that 100 per cent mortality was only obtained in controls for animals receiving more than 10^3 leukaemic cells; the animals who only received 10^2 cells did not have greater than 60 per cent mortality.

None of the three treatments was effective in the animals that received 10^7 or 10^6 leukaemic cells; on the other hand, BCG and the vaccination with irradiated tumour cells and the association of these two treatments gave only an increase of the mean survival time and a cure of a certain number of the animals in the 4 groups of mice who had received less than 10^5 leukaemic cells.

Table 1 shows a resume of these results and a statistical analysis.

Table 1. *Statistical analysis of the difference of survival of treated groups of animals compared to the controls (p. values)*

Number of leukaemic cells grafted to induce the leukaemias	10^7	10^6	10^5	10^4	10^3	10^2
B.C.G.	0	0	0.1	0.1	0.1	0.1
B.C.G. + irradiated leukaemic cells	0	0	0.1	0.1	0.1	0.1
Irradiated leukaemic cells	0	0	0.1	0.1	0.1	NS

This experiment also shows that the combination of repeated BCG and the administration of a single injection of irradiated leukaemic cells was more effective against the leukaemia than the administration of BCG alone, or of irradiated leukaemic cells, when the number of grafted leukaemic cells was 10^5. This difference was very significant at the 30th day: $p < 1$ per cent.

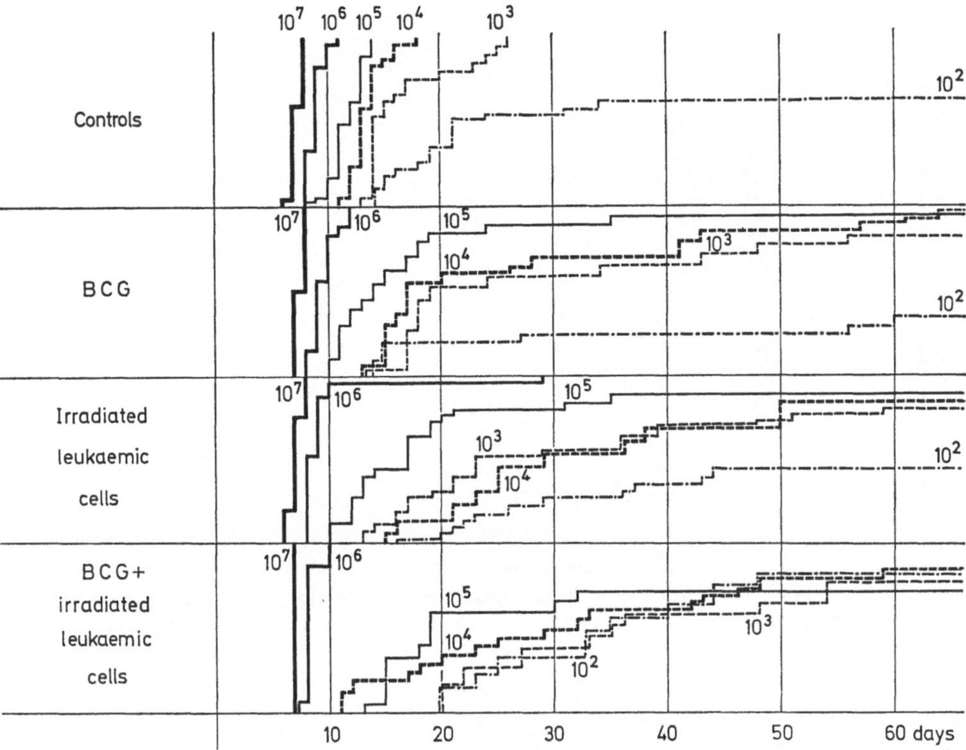

Fig. 6. Cumulative survival of mice grafted with 10^2 to 10^7 L 1210 leukaemia cells: not treated or treated in the 24 hours following the graft by BCG, or irradiated leukaemic cells, or association of BCG and leukaemic cells

Discussion

It was known that the administration, *before* the graft of a tumour, of adjuvants [2, 4, 10] or of inactivated tumour cells [1], can inhibit the growth of the tumour. Active immunotherapy was only conceived as a method of preventive therapy, such as in the case of infectious diseases. But preventive active immunotherapy is outside any therapeutic, clinical application, because of the ignorance of tumour antigens in human cancers.

The experiments reported in this work demonstrate the possible curative action of active immunotherapy against an established experimental tumour.

The L 1210 leukaemia was grafted into F1 hybrid animals and makes it likely that allogeneic inhibition effects [11] were probably associated with the inhibition caused by the immunisation. Choquet and Malaise [12], working in this laboratory, have shown that allogeneic inhibition is certainly present when L 1210 leukaemic cells are grafted into hybrid (C57Bl/6×DBA/2) F1 mice, but the degree of inhibition is minor in relation to that caused by the immunisation. The control animals in our experiments enabled us to avoid attributing to immunisation any effect that may have arisen from allogeneic inhibition.

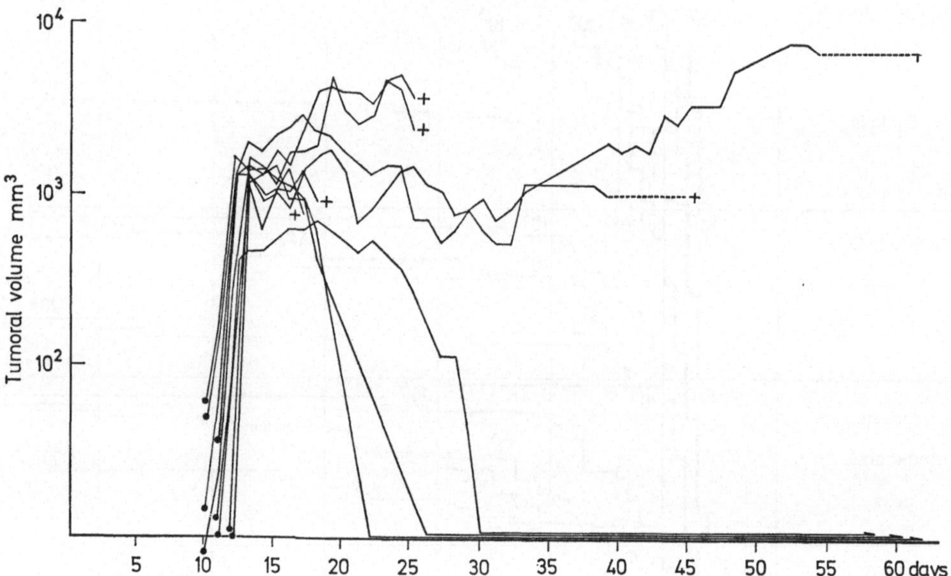

Fig. 7. Tumoral volume of each mouse in the group of mice carrying L 1210 leukaemia and treated by the association of BCG and irradiated leukaemic cells 24 h after the graft

L 1210 leukaemia is a leukaemia which has passed hosts by successive grafting, and it can be questioned whether the leukaemic cells might have lost their tumour antigens; a study by Motta [13] has shown that, though these antigens are feeble, they are still present in the cells.

Finally, it may be questioned if the immune effects obtained arise from these tumour antigens or from histocompatibility antigens bound to mutations sustained either by the leukaemia or by the DBA/2 line which forms part of the constitution of the F1 hybrid. One can reply that, if histocompatibility antigens exist on the leukaemic cells that are not carried by the recipient mice, they are certainly very weak, for all grafts of this leukaemia kill 100 per cent of the recipients when 10^3 or more tumour cells are given, and the animals are killed within 11 days once 10^6 cells have been injected. Hence, if histocompatibility antigens do exist, then they can only act as very feeble antigens, with a force not greater than those of the tumour antigens. It is reasonable to hope that the conclusions reached in the present study can be applied to the leukaemias whose only antigenic difference compared to the host, is due to their tumour antigens.

The first major concept that comes from these experiments is the power of active immunotherapy to eradicate leukaemia. Fig. 3 shows that 50 per cent of the mice treated with a combination of BCG and irradiated leukaemic cells were cured, and Fig. 7, which gives an overall analysis of an experiment and shows the growth of the tumour volume in each mouse, demonstrates that this therapy is also able to cause the regression of an established tumour. Though many chemotherapeutic drugs are capable of delaying the mortality of mice carrying L 1210 leukaemia (see 14), few are capable of curing 50 per cent of the treated animals, and causing the volume of an established tumour to regress, in the manner that was achieved with active immunotherapy in these experiments.

This power to eradicate leukaemia and to effect a cure, suggests that active immunotherapy is capable of destroying all the cells in a cancer population. This is in contrast to chemotherapy, which obeys first-order kinetics [15].

Two reservations to these concepts should be considered at this point: a) in two mice out of 150 animals which survived to the sixtieth day after a graft of leukaemia, very late relapses occured after 120 and 180 days respectively (these 150 animals were in part from the experiments described above, as well as from other experiments); these two relapses occured in animals that were thought to have been cured; b) though immunotherapy is capable of eradicating an entire tumour population in the majority of the animals that have been treated, it is only capable of doing this if the population is relatively small. In the case of L 1210 leukaemia in the mouse, only when the number of tumour cells is not greater than 10^5. SKIPPER and his colleagues [15] have shown that mice carying L 1210 leukaemia, and cured by the administration of cyclophosphamide, are insensitive to a new graft of this leukaemia, owing to an immunisation against the graft, but this only occured when the number of tumour cells inoculated was not greater than 10^5.

It will be seen that the pattern of tumour growth was according to a gompertz function, consisting of two phases, rapid then slow, and immunotherapy only acted upon the slow phase: 1) in some instances, immunotherapy reduces the slope of this part of the growth phase; in this case, it only slightly delays the mortality; 2) in other animals, the slope of this second phase descends, the tumour regresses and the animal is cured; 3) finally, in other animals, this slope is replaced by a plateau, associated with a considerable delay of the mortality, sometimes to as long as a month, which is very considerable for L 1210 leukaemia: this observation, as well as the two very late relapses mentioned above, poses the question wether active immunotherapy may be capable of arresting and maintaining cells at Go for a long period; nevertheless, a study in progress [16], which is based on the cytophotometric examination of the cells of tumors the growth of which is represented by a plateau, suggests that, on the contrary, it acts essentially on the cell loss coefficient, it does not prolong the cycle and it does not increase the percentage of cells in Go.

From a practical point of view, it is convenient to stress that the repetition of the administration of BCG, the best of the adjuvants in his study, has a better curative effect than giving a single dose (but there is a slight increase in the mortality), whilst a single injection or irradiated cells is just as effective as repeated injections. BCG is more effective than irradiated cells when its administration is commenced before the graft of the leukaemia. A single injection of irradiated cells is more effective when they are given after the graft of the tumour than when they are given beforehand. But, in both these instances, there is another important, practical conclusion: the combination of BCG and the irradiated leukaemic cells has a better effect at any of the time periods compared to when these stimuli are given alone (Fig. 2, 3, 4, 5).

This signifies that neither of these two treatments can induce a maximal stimulatory effect and that it is likely that they act upon two different systems. This has led us to suggests to recommend in clinical practice, the use of the combination of an adjuvant with a specific vaccine.

MATHÉ and his colleagues [17, 18] have recently published the results of a clinical trial, in which immunotherapy was used. The number of leukaemic cells was reduced to a level as low as possible, at first by chemotherapy to induce a remission, then by complementary chemotherapy, using sequentially all the drugs that are known to be effective against acute lymphoblastic leukaemia. The results of this clinical trial, which have been based upon the results of the experiments discussed in this paper, have been encouraging. Ten control patients treated by the chemotherapeutic regime and then receiving no further therapy, all relapsed within 130 days, following the arrest of chemotherapy; 12 patients of the 20 treated by active immunotherapy, consisting of either the application of BCG, or the vaccination with irradiated leukaemic cells, or a combination of these two treatments, had not relapsed by 130 days. Seven of these patients have still not relapsed up to the present day: for one of them, this is more than 3 years and a half; for 2, a period of more than 2 years and a half, and for 4 others, periods of more than one year and a half, since stopping chemotherapy.

Summary

1. In the first experiment, a comparison was made of the effects of BCG, Corynebacterium parvum, Mycobacterium cheiloni, Bordetella pertussis or irradiated leukaemic cells, administrated once or several times *after* the graft of 10^4 L 1210 leukaemic cells. Out of the adjuvants, BCG was the only one with any notable effect, and repeated administration was more active than when given as a single dose; the irradiated leukaemic cells were more active than BCG, and had identical activity whether they were injected once or repeatedly.

2. In the second experiment, a comparison was made of the effects of BCG, of irradiated leukaemic cells and a combination of them both, according to the time of their administration in relation to a graft of 10^4 L 1210 leukaemic cells. The BCG was given as repeated doses, whilst the irradiated leukaemic cells in the form of a single dose. The BCG was more active than the irradiated leukaemic cells when they were administered before the graft of the leukaemia; the irradiated leukaemic cells were more active when they were given after the graft of the leukaemia. A combination of the two forms of immunotherapy was more active than BCG alone, even when this was administered before the graft of the leukaemia, and more active than the irradiated leukaemic cells, even when they were administered after the graft of the leukaemia.

3. In the third experiment, (C57Bl/6×DBA/2) F1 mice were grafted with a variable number of L 1210 (DBA/2) leukaemic cells; they were treated during the 24 hours which followed this graft, by active immunotherapy, either non-specific, using BCG, or specific, using leukaemic cells that had been irradiated at 15,000 rads, or a combination of both of these stimuli. The three procedures were confirmed not only to be capable of prolonging the survival of the mice but also curing a considerable number of them. But cure was only obtained in those groups of animals in whom the number of grafted cells was 10^5 or fewer. When larger numbers of leukaemic cells were grafted, these treatments were found to be ineffective.

4. The possible clinical application of these findings is discussed. They have already been applied to a trial of active immunotherapy for the treatment of acute lymphoblastic leukaemia in man, and have shown that such a therapy can be effective.

References

1. Glynn, J. P., Humphreys, S. R., Trivers, G., Bianco, A. R., Goldin, A.: Studies on immunity to leukaemia L 1210 in mice. Cancer Res. 23, 1008 (1963).
2. Amiel, J. L.: Immunotherapie active non spécifique par le BCG de la leucémie virale E♂G2 chez des receveurs isogéniques. Rev. franç. Étud. clin. biol. 12, 912 (1967).
3. Balner, H., Old, L. J., Clarke, D. A.: Accelerated rejection of male skin isografts by female C57Bl/6 mice infected with BCG. Proc. Soc. exp. Biol. (N. Y.) 109, 58 (1962).

4. Biozzi, G., Stiffel, C., Halpern, B. N., Mouton, D.: Effect of inoculation with BCG on the development of Ehrlich ascites tumor in the mouse. C. R. Soc. Biol. (Paris) **153**, 987 (1959).
5. Halpern, B. N., Biozzi, G., Stiffel, C., Mouton, D.: Effect of stimulation on the reticulo-endothelial system by inoculation of the BCG on the development of the atypical Guerin T-S epithelioma in the rat C. R. Soc. Biol. (Paris) **153**, 919 (1959).
6. — Prevot, A. R., Biozzi, G., Stiffel, C., Mouton, D., Morard, J. C., Bouthillier, Y., Decreusefond, C.: Stimulation de l'activité phagocytaire du système réticulo-endothélial provoquée par Corynebacterium parvum. J. Rétic.-Endoth. Soc. **1**, 73 (1964).
7. — Biozzi, G., Stiffel, C., Mouton, D.: Inhibition of tumor growth by administration of killed Corynebacterium parvum. Nature (Lond.) **212**, 853 (1966).
8. Woodruff, M. F. A., Boak, J. L.: Inhibitory effect of injection of Corynebacterium parvum on the growth of tumour transplants in isogenic hosts. Brit. J. Cancer **20**, 345 (1966).
9. Mathé, G.: Immunothérapie de la L 1210 administrée après la greffe tumorale. Rev. franç. Étud. clin. biol. **13**, 881 (1968).
10. Old, L. J., Clarke, D. A., Benacerraf, B.: Effect of bacillus Calmette-Guérin (BCG) infection of transplanted tumours in the mouse. Nature (Lond.) **184**, 291 (1959).
11. Möller, G.: Antibody induced depression of the immune response: a study of the mechanisms in various systems. Transplantation **2**, 405 (1964).
12. Choquet, C., Malaise, E.: Allogenic inhibition and kinetics of L 1210 leukaemia. To be published.
13. Motta, R.: The passive immunotherapy of murine leukaemia. I. The production of antisera against leukaemic neonatigens. Rev. Europ. Étud. clin. biol. **15**, 161 (1970).
14. Mathé, G., Schwarzenberg, L., Hayat, M., Schneider, M.: Chimiothérapie de la leucémie L 1210: comparaison pour 7 composés, des effects de l'administration continue sur 20 jours et de l'administration d'une dose unique massive, précoce ou tardive. Rev. franç. Étud. clin. biol. **13**, 951 (1968).
15. Skipper, E., Schabel, F. M., Wilcox, W. S.: Experimental evaluation of potential anticancer agents. XIII. On the criteria and kinetics associated with "curability" of experimental leukemia. Cancer Chemother. Rep. **35**, 3 (1964).
16. Bulens, C., Lheritier, J., Mathé, G.: To be published.
17. Mathé, G., Amiel, J. L., Schwarzenberg, L., Schneider, M., Cattan, A., Schlumberger, J. R., Hayat, M., de Vassal, F.: Démonstration de l'efficacité de l'immunothérapie active dans la leucémie aigue lymphoblastique humaine. Rev. franç. Étud. clin. biol. **13**, 454 (1968).
18. — — — — — — — — Active immunotherapy for acute lymphoblastic leukaemia. Lancet **1969 I**, 697.

Experimental Basis and Clinical Results of Leukemia Adoptive Immunotherapy

G. Mathé, L. Schwarzenberg, J. L. Amiel, P. Pouillart, M. Schneider, and A. Cattan

Institut de Cancérologie et d'Immunogénétique, Hôpital Paul-Brousse, 14, Avenue Paul-Vaillant-Couturier, 94-Villejuif

With 5 Figures

Adoptive immunotherapy of cancer is based on the lytic effect on tumor cells of lymphocytes either transfused or produced by a bone marrow graft. In both conditions one can consider two possibilities according to if the donor is immunized (specific adoptive immunotherapy) or is not immunized (non specific adoptive immunotherapy) against the tumor associated antigens.

1. Lymphocyte Transfusions

In the case of allogeneic lymphocyte transfusions, without any immunological conditionning of the recipient, one can expect only a short term effect. But among the parameters which condition the antileukaemia effect of lymphocyte transfusions, two of them seemed to be worthwhile to be studied: the number of lymphocytes for a given number of tumor cells and immunization of the donor, Alexander (1968) having obtained remarkable antitumor effects with lymphocytes from immunized donors.

The following experiment (Mathé and Pouillart, 1970) has been performed to get precise information of these two parameters.

AkR mice, 2 months old, received injections of 10^6 K36 leukaemic cells; K36 leukaemia is a grafted leukaemia originated from a spontaneous AkR leukaemia. These mice were treated by intravenous injections of either 10^4 or 10^6 allogeneic lymphocytes, the donors being C57Bl/6 mice, not immunized or immunized with irradiated cells from E ♂ G2 leukaemia, which is a leukaemia induced in C57Bl/6 mice by Gross virus, which in other words, is carrying the same tumor associated antigens as K36 leukaemia.

The results of this experiment are shown on Fig. 1. One can see that no benefit is obtained from 10^4 lymphocytes from normal C57Bl/6 mice, while a substantial and identical antileukaemic effect is obtained from either 10^6 lymphocytes from normal C57Bl/6 mice or 10^4 lymphocytes from C57Bl/6 mice immunized against leukaemia associated antigens. A more dramatic effect is obtained with 10^6 lymphocytes from C57Bl/6 mice immunized against leukaemia associated antigens.

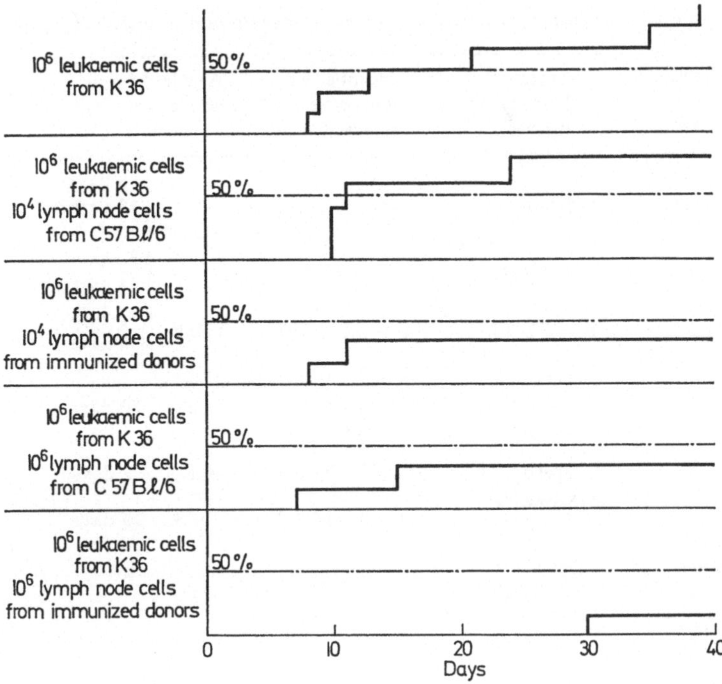

Fig. 1. Adoptive immunotherapy of K36 AkR leukaemia by C57Bl/6 lymph node cells. The better therapeutic effect is obtained with lymph node cells immunized with E ♂ G2 leukaemia

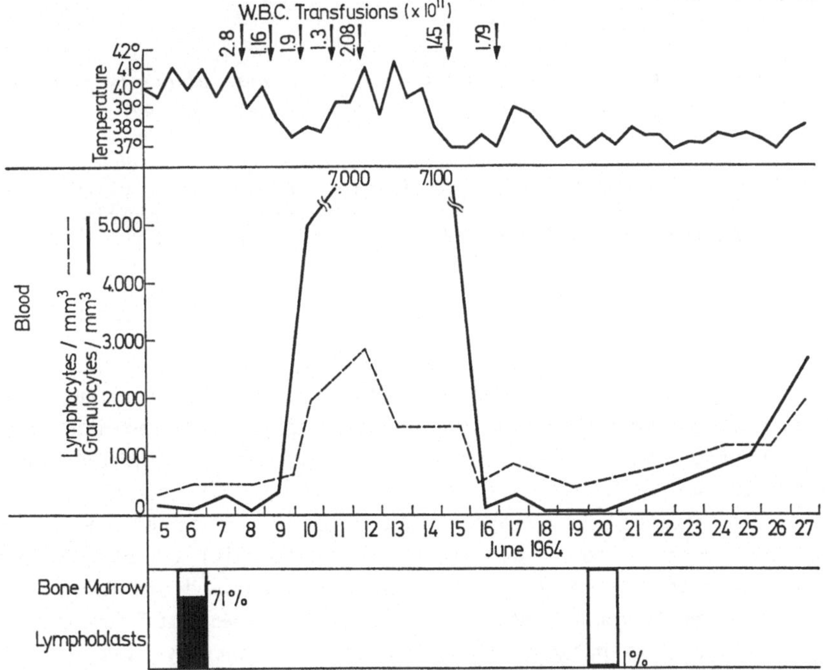

Fig. 2. Induction of a remission in a patient with acute lymphoblastic leukaemia by leucocyte transfusions from donors with chronic myelocytic leukaemia

Table 1. *Transfusion of leucocytes from allogeneic non immunized donors*

Type of leukaemia	State of leucocytes injected	Number of leucocytes injected	Antileukaemic effect		Signs of secondary syndrome
Lymphoblastic 14	Fresh	1×10^{11} to 1.2×10^{12}	5 CR[a]	8 days	[a]
				15 days	
	Incubated at 37° C	6×10^{11} to 9.8×10^{11}		20 days	[a]
				80 days	[a]
				4 months	[a]
	Stored at −70° C	9×10^{10} to 5.0×10^{11}	2 ICR	7 days	[a]
				8 days	
Myeloblastic 3	Fresh	9.4×10^{11}			
	Stored at −70° C	1×10^{11}	1 CR	10 days	
		3.5×10^{11}			
Monoblastic 2	Fresh	7.1×10^{11}	1 CR	7 days	[a b]
	Stored at −70° C	8×10^{10}	1 ICR	15 days	
Histiocytomonocytic 1	Stored at −70° C	6.3×10^{10}		0	
Acute leukaemic syndrome secondary to a lymphosarcoma	Stored at −70° C	1×10^{11}		0	[a]

[a] = One associated with Vincristine.
[b] = Cutaneous signs absent.

Table 2. *The immunotherapeutic effect of leucocyte transfusions. Relation between the antileukaemic action and the existence of a secondary syndrom*

	Complete remissions	Incomplete remissions	No effect
Secondary syndrome present	4	2	1
Absence of the signs of a secondary syndrome	1	2	11

Hence these two parameters which were studied in the experiment, the number of lymphocytes transfused and specific immunization against tumor associated antigens are both important, the first being the only one which can be considered in clinical practice at present.

Our clinical practice with lymphocyte transfusions has confirmed their efficiency, namely their capacity to induce short but (apparently) complete remissions (SCHWARZENBERG et al., 1966, 1968, 1968). The results obtained with chronic myelocytic leukaemia leucocytes, are shown in Table 1; one can see that 7 complete remissions were obtained in patients resistant to any chemotherapy. Fig. 2 gives an example of such a remission, and Table 2 shows the correlation between the appearance of the graft versus host manifestations and the antileukaemic effect; the good

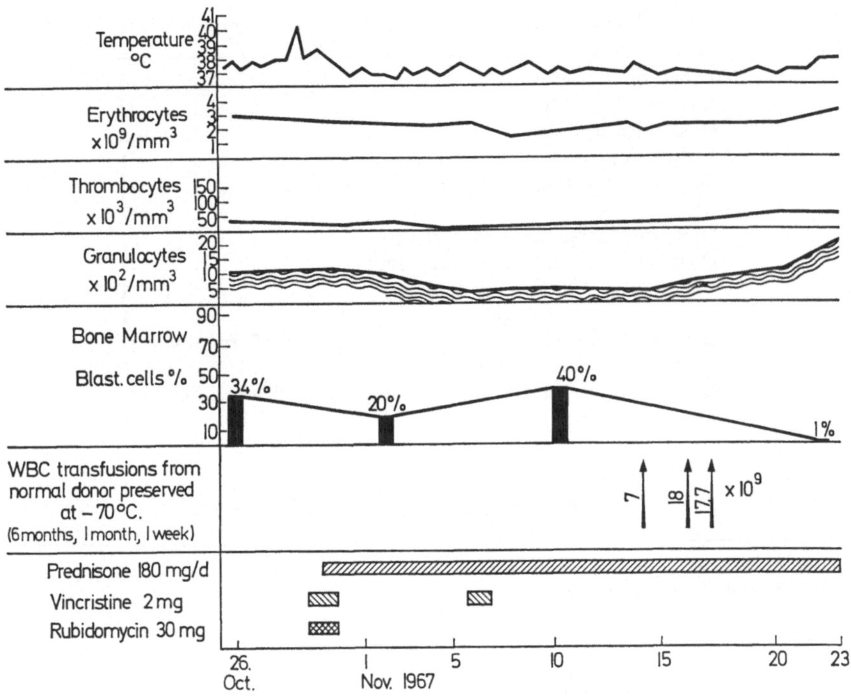

Fig. 3. Induction of a remission in a patient with acute lymphoblastic leukaemia by leucocyte transfusions from normal donor

correlation is strongly in favour of the immunological mechanisms for the induction of these remissions.

Since we have been working with the IBM continuous flow blood cell separator, we have been treating 9 patients with acute leukaemia resistant to any chemotherapy by pure lymphocyte preparations (obtained from normal donors) and we have obtained 2 "complete remissions". Fig. 3 shows an example.

2. Bone Marrow Transplantation

From lymphocyte transfusions in patients not immunosuppressed, one can only expect a short term effect, because the lymphocytes transfused are destroyed by the immune reactions of the host. To get a permanent effect, one has theoretically to graft the tissue which produces lymphocytes, namely bone marrow. We have not performed any recent experiment on adoptive immunotherapy based on bone marrow grafting and we shall only recall the principle of the therapeutic method based on experiments we performed some years ago on a L 1210 grafted leukaemia (MATHÉ and BERNARD, 1959; MATHÉ, AMIEL, NIEMETZ, 1962; MATHÉ and SCHWARZENBERG, 1968), a virus induced leukaemia (Charlotte Friend leukaemia) (MATHÉ, AMIEL and FRIEND, 1962; MATHÉ and AMIEL, 1964), and a virus spontaneous leukaemia (AkR leukaemia) (MATHÉ and BERNARD, 1958; MATHÉ, AMIEL and BERNARD, 1960). These experiments showed that if one has a subject (A), carrying leukaemic cells (a), the leukaemia having being possibly induced by a virus (α), if we graft bone marrow

Table 3. *Results of graft attempts after total body irradiation*

Number of attempts	24
Failure of the graft	7
Died with aplasia	5
Failure followed by isogenic restoration	1
Survival in aplasia until relapse of leukemia	1
Grafts	17
Died with acute secondary syndrome	10
Died with subacute secondary syndrome	2
(Candida albicans septicaemia)	1
(Varicella encephalitis)	1
Died with chronic secondary syndrome at 20 months (herpes zoster encephalitis)	1
Complicated by a controlled secondary syndrome, died with leukaemia	4

Table 4. *Evidence of the graft*

Erythrocytic antigens [a]
Sex-linked granulocyte appendices [b]
Mononuclear sex chromatin [c]
Sex chromosomes [d]
Groups of immunoglobulins (Inv) [d]
Specific immune tolerance based on the chimerism [d]

[a] Mathé, Jammet, Pendic, Schwarzenberg et al., 1959.
[b] Mathé, Bernard, de Vries et al., 1960.
[c] Seman, 1961.
[d] Mathé, Amiel, Schwarzenberg, Cattan, Schneider et al., 1963.

(B) after a total body irradiation at a lethal dose which not only conditions the recipient for the take of the graft, but reduces considerably the number of the tumour cells, the reaction of the lymphocytes produced by the bone marrow (B) against leukaemic cells (a) is able to eradicate the cells which escape irradiation; the reaction of these lymphocytes against the virus (α) is able to reduce its quantity and, if some virus (α) persists, one may hope that it may not be able to induce a new leukaemia in the hemopoietic cells (B) if 100% of the bone marrow cells are (B).

The data acquired in 10 years practice with bone marrow grafted leukaemia patients prepared (for immunosuppression and leukaemic cell reduction) by total body irradiation, are confirming the value of this therapeutical method.

Table 3 shows the incidence of the secondary disease and summaries our experience with the allogeneic bone marrow grafting in man (Mathé et al., 1959, 1960, 1963, 1965, 1968). The positive take of the bone marrow graft has been proved by the various tests listed in Table 4. The anti-leukaemic effect has been analysed by the study of four cases (Fig. 4), where the patients have survived the secondary disease. In three of them, the graft was only partial and transitory: only 50 per cent of the red blood cells were produced by the graft; the graft survived for about three months in these three patients. A "complete remission", lasting for nine months was obtained in the first patient, and for five months and six months respectively in the

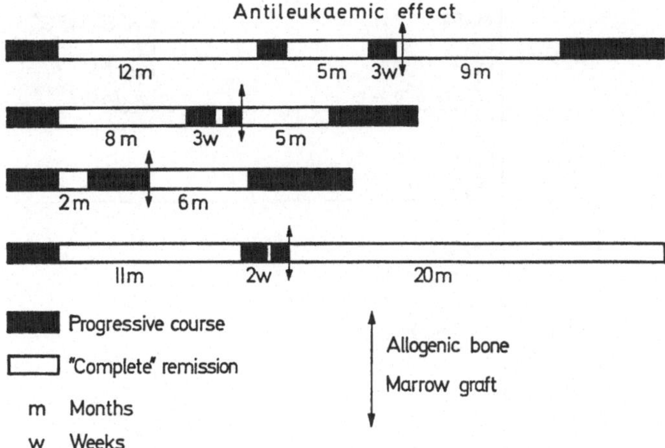

Fig. 4. The active phases and remissions in 4 patients treated by allogeneic bone marrow grafts and who had not died from bone marrow aplasia or from secondary syndrome

second and the third. In the fourth patient, the graft was total and seemed to be definite, in as much as, when the patient died twenty months after the grafting, from a herpes encephalitis, an infectious complication of the immune deficiency that was related to a latent secondary disease, 100% of the red cells were produced by the graft; at the time of death, 20 months after the graft, he was still in complete remission and, at autopsy, no leukaemic cells were demonstrated in any of this tissues.

It is very difficult to control the secondary disease in allogeneic haemopoietic radio-chimeras, because of their frequent infections.

Though we know that the secondary disease is due to the reaction of the grafted lymphoid cells against the recipient's antigen, we known this complication is even more severe when the dose of the irradiation is higher. Hence the idea of replacing acute total body irradiation by some means of immunological conditioning which would favorise less the secondary disease. While GEORGES SANTOS group in Baltimore (1969) is working on cyclophosphamide, we have been following a research

Table 5. *Attempt of bone marrow graft after conditionning by antilymphocytic serum*

	Number of cases	Take of the graft
Acute leukaemias in visible phase of the disease		
Non aplastic	4	0
Aplastic	3	2
Acute leukaemias in non visible phase of the disease		
Aplastic	2	2
Thalassaemia	1	0
Idiopathic medullar aplasia	2	0

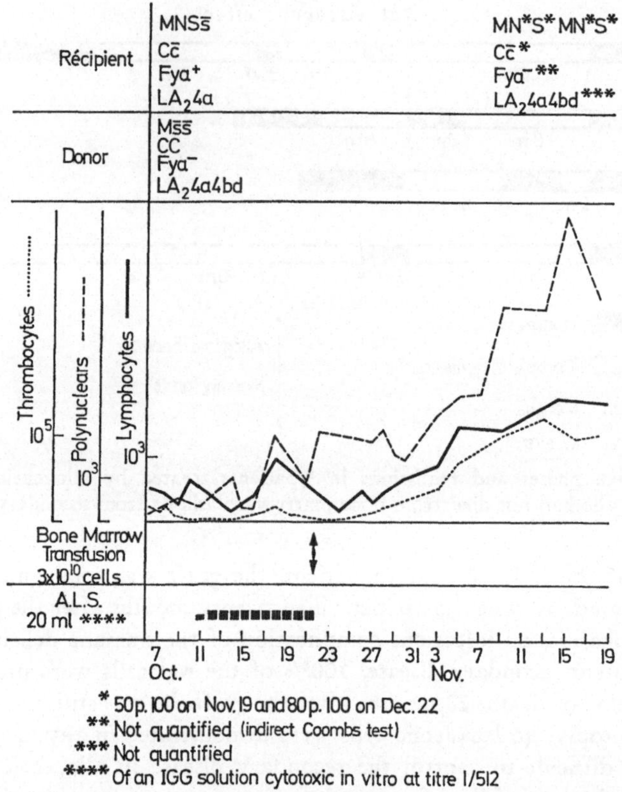

Fig. 5. Allogeneic bone marrow graft in man after conditioning donor and recipient by antilymphocyte serum

protocol in which the preparation of the recipient is assured by horse anti-human lymphocyte serum (IgG) (Mathé et al., 1968) administered to the donor and the recipient for one trial out of 2 and to the recipient alone for the other one. The results are summarized on Table 5, which shows that the incidence of the take is not rare in patients whose bone marrow was aplastic. Fig. 5 shows an example of such a take. The secondary disease is very discrete but at the same time the antileukaemic effect of the bone marrow seems poor, may be because of the paralysis by ALS of the donor lymphocytes, may be because of the antileukaemic effect related to the reaction of the grafted lymphocytes can only be effective if the number of the tumor cells is low at the time of the graft, which was realized by the conditioning by total body irradiation and which suggests to adopt a protocol in which ALS would be preceded either by the administration of a cytostatic substance (for the destruction of leukaemic cells), or by repeated small doses of total body irradiation.

Summary

Adoptive immunotherapy of leukaemia is based on the lytic effect on tumour cells of lymphocytes either transfused or produced by a bone marrow graft.

In the case of allogeneic lymphocyte transfusions, without any immunological conditioning of the host, one can except only a short time effect. The experiment described in mice shows that this effect can nevertheless be strong if the number of lymphocytes transfused is high, or if the donor is immunized against the tumour-associated antigens. Trials in man have demonstrated the possibility of obtaining short remissions in acute leukaemia, either with leucocytes obtained from CML donors or from normal donors (isolated with the IBM blood cell separator).

In the case of bone marrow graft, remissions of average duration were obtained when the graft was transitory; a remission of more than 20 months has been obtained in a patient whose graft was permanent; no sign of leukaemia was found at autopsy when he died from an infectious complication of the graft-versus-host reaction.

References

Alexander, P.: Immunotherapy of cancer: experiments with primary tumour and syngeneic tumour grafts. Progr. exp. Tumor Res. (Basel) **10**, 22 (1968).

Mathé, G., Amiel, J. L.: Réduction de la concentration plasmatique du virus Charlotte Friend par immunothérapie adoptive. C. R. Acad. Sci. (Paris) **259**, 4408 (1964).

— — Bernard, J.: Traitement de souris AkR à l'âge de 6 mois par irradiation totale suivie de transfusions de cellules hématopoïétiques homologues. Incidences respectives de la leucémie et du syndrome secondaire. Bull. Cancer **47**, 331 (1960).

— — Friend, Ch.: Essai de traitement de la leucémie de Charlotte Friend par la greffe de cellules hématopoïétiques de donneurs vaccinés. Bull. Cancer **49**, 416 (1962).

— — Niemetz, J.: Greffe de moelle osseuse après irradiation totale chez des souris leucémiques suivie de l'administration d'un produit antimitotique pour réduire la fréquence du syndrome secondaire et ajouter à l'effet antileucémique. C. R. Acad. Sci. (Paris) **54**, 3603 (1962).

— — Schwarzenberg, L.: Bone marrow transplantation. In: Human transplantation, Vol. 1. New York: Grune and Stratton 1968, p. 284.

— — — Cattan, A., Schneider, M.: Haemopoietic chimera in man after allogeneic (homologous) bone marrow transplantation: control of the secondary syndrome, specific tolerance due to the chimerism. Brit. med. J. **2**, 1633 (1963).

— — — — — Vries, M. J. de, Tubiana, M., Lalanne, C., Binet, J. L., Papiernik, M., Seman, G., Matsukura, M., Mery, A. M., Schwarzmann, V., Flaisler, A.: Successful allogeneic bone marrow transplantation in man: chimerism induced specific tolerance and possible antileukaemic effects. Blood **25**, 179 (1965).

— — — Schneider, M., Cattan, A., Schlumberger, J. R., Hayat, M., Vassal, F. de, Jasmin, C., Rosenfeld, C., Choay, J., Trolard, P.: Greffe de moelle osseuse allogénique chez l'homme prouvée par six marqueurs antigéniques après conditionnement du receveur et du donneur par le sérum antilymphocytaire. Rev. franç. Étud. clin. biol. **13**, 1025 (1968).

— Bernard, J.: Essai de traitement par l'irradiation X suivie de greffe de cellules myéloïdes homologues de souris atteintes de leucémie spontanée très avancée. Bull. Cancer **45**, 289 (1958).

— — Essai de traitement de la leucémie L 1210 par l'irradiation X suivie de transfusions de cellules hématopoïétiques normales (isologues ou homologues, lymphoïdes ou myéloïdes adultes ou embryonnaires). Rev. franç. Étud. clin. biol. **4**, 442 (1959).

— — Schwarzenberg, L., Larrieu, M. J., Lalanne, C., Dutreix, A., Denoix, P., Surmont, J., Schwarzmann, V., Coeara, B.: Essai de traitement de sujets atteints de leucémie aigue en rémission par irradiation totale suivie de transfusion de moelle osseuse homologue. Rev. franç. Étud. clin. biol. **4**, 675 (1959).

— — Vries, M. J. de, Schwarzenberg, L., Larrieu, M. J., Lalanne, C., Dutreix, A., Amiel, J. L., Surmont, J.: Nouveaux essais de greffe de moelle osseuse homologue après irradiation totale chez des enfants atteints de leucémie aigue en rémission. Le problème du syndrome secondaire chez l'homme. Rev. Hémat. **115**, 15 (1960).

— Pouillart, P.: Transfusions of lymphocytes from non immunized or immunized donors in mice leukaemia therapy. In: Internat. Symp. of the C.N.R.S. on white blood cell transfusions, Paris 1969. C.N.R.S. (in press).

MATHÉ, G., SCHWARZENBERG, L.: Immunothérapie adoptive locale de la leucémie L 1210 ascitique. Analyse des facteurs de son efficacité. Europ. J. Cancer 4, 22 (1968).

SANTOS, G. W.: Preparation of a recipient for a transplant by cyclophosphamide. Comm. Symp. on "bone marrow transplantation". Paris 1969.

SCHWARZENBERG, L., MATHÉ, G., AMIEL, J. L., CATTAN, A., SCHNEIDER, M., SCHLUMBERGER, J. R.: Adoptive immunotherapy by transfusions of leucocytes. Lancet 2, 365 (1966).

— — GROUCHY, J. DE, NAVA, C. DE, VRIES, M. J. DE, AMIEL, J. L., CATTAN, A., SCHNEIDER, M., SCHLUMBERGER, J. R.: White blood cell transfusions. Israel J. med. Sci. 1, 925 (1965).

— NAGI, M. S., PRADET-BALADE, O., MATHÉ, G.: Utilisation pour la séparation des lymphocytes sanguins du séparateur de cellules sanguines à débit continu. Nouv. Rev. franç. Hémat. 8, 579 (1968).

II. Strategy of the Treatment

Remission Induction in Adults with Acute Myelogenous Leukemia

E. J. Freireich, G. P. Bodey, S. Hart, V. Rodriguez, J. P. Whitecar, and E. Frei, III

University of Texas M. D. Anderson Hospital and Tumor Institute Houston, Texas

Introduction

Major progress has been achieved in the chemotherapy of acute lymphocytic leukemia. In general the sequence of progress in this disease has been as follows: production of complete remission; increase of the complete remission rate to greater than 70% of patients with combination therapy; demonstration that maintained remissions are longer than unmaintained remissions; increase in duration of remissions by intensive treatment, combination therapy, optimized dose schedules, cyclic therapy, and intermittent reinduction; and substantial increase in survival [1, 2, 3, 4, 5, 6, 7, 8, 9]. Progress in the treatment of adults with acute myelogenous leukemia has lagged. While there are a few agents capable of producing complete remission in a minority of patients, remission induction programs capable of producing complete remission in the majority of patients have yet to be defined. This article will describe our efforts over the past three years to improve the complete remission rate in adult acute myelogenous leukemia.

Methods

The programs that have been most effective in producing complete remissions are listed in Table 1. In addition to these programs we have studied a number of new agents such as dimethylaminoimidazole carboxamide triazeno, methyl mercaptopurine riboside (MMPR) and L-asparaginase. These new agents have produced remission rates of less than 15% and will not be included in this analysis. The doses and schedules for the major programs are included in Table 1. Note that for the most part treatment has been given in intermittent courses rather than continuously. This is based on definitive evidence in experimental *in vivo* systems and selected clinical evidence which indicates that intermittent intensive treatment is superior to continuous treatment in the rapidly proliferating tumors [10, 11, 12].

Table 1. *Treatment programs and rational*

Treatment programs	Dose route and schedule	Rationale
MP	90 mg/M²/d p. o.	Activity in S 180
MP + MMPR	MP 300 mg/M²/d×5 i. v. MMPR 100 mg/M²/d×5 i. v. 5 day courses every 2 wks.	No cross resistance and synergism in L 1210 and Ehrlich
Ara-C	200 mg/M²/day by continuous infusion. 5 day courses every 2 wks.	Intermittent courses more active in L 1210
Ara-C + Cyclo.	Ara-C and cyclo. 150 mg/M²/d for 4 days (given i. v. q 8 hrs). 4 day courses every 2 wks.	Synergism between alkylating agents and Ara-C in experimental system
COAP	Cytoxan and Ara-C as above plus Prednisone and Oncovin (vincristine)	See text

Table 2. *Acute myelocytic leukemia in adults: remission induction by treatment program*

Patient categories	MP [a]	MP + MMPR	Ara-C	Ara-C + Cyclophos.	COAP [b]
Time of study	1958—1960	1966—1967	1966—1967	1967—1968	1968—
Total entered	31	34	16	32	19
Adequate trial [c]	14	18	11	27	14
Adequate trial/ total entered	45%	53%	69%	84%	74%
Complete remission (CR)	3	8	5	13	10
CR/Adequate trial	21%	44%	45%	48%	71%
CR/Total entered	9%	24%	31%	41%	53%

[a] From ALGB. Blood 18, 431 (1961).
[b] COAP = Cyclophosphamide, vincristine, Ara-C, prednisone (ongoing).
[c] Adequate Trial-6 or more weeks of treatment.

Results

Response to remission induction therapy is presented in Table 2. The agent which has been most commonly employed for remission induction in AML is 6-mercaptopurine (MP). The data included under MP in Table 2 was obtained from a multi-institute study performed between 1958 and 1960 [13]. It generally takes up to 6 weeks for patients to achieve a bone marrow complete remission (less than 10% blast and promyelocytes). Thus an adequate trial is defined as 6 or more weeks of treatment. For MP only 45% of patients had an adequate trial. The fraction of patients with adequate trials has increased over the past five years and for the two programs (ara-C + Cytoxan and COAP) in excess of 70% of patients received an adequate trial.

Factors which influence the fraction of patients receiving adequate trial are given in Table 3. Good prognostic features in patient selection and the availability and

Table 3. *Adequate trial adequate trials/total entered patient selection (youth, low WBC etc.) × supportive care toxicity*

Treatment		MP	MP+ MMPR	Ara-C	Ara-C + cyt	COAP
Years		1958—1960	1966—1967	1966—1967	1967—1968	1968—
Patients age (median)		—	56	42	51	55
Toxicity [a]	Marrow	2+	3+	4+	4+	4+
	GI	2+	3+	1+	1+	1+
Supportive care			Platelets →	→	→	→
				Life island →	→	→
					Laminar air →	→
						Carbenicillin →

[a] Toxicity — 0—4 + Scale.

application of supportive care favorably affect the proportion of adequate trials whereas toxicity, particularly myelotoxicity, adversely affects the proportion of adequate trials. The major patient selection factor is age; the older patients are less responsive. The median age in years for the various treatment programs is essentially the same with the possible exception of the ara-C program (Table 3). The myelosuppressive effects of the given programs have increased in recent years (Table 3). Increasing myelosuppression would, of itself, decrease the fraction of adequate trials. The fact that the opposite has happened is a tribute to major improvements in supportive care. Some of the factors involved in supportive care and the approximate time of introduction are given in Table 3. It is to be emphasized that supportive care has improved over a very broad clinical base and that only selected factors are included in Table 3.

The observation that 6-methylmercaptopurine riboside (MMPR) was not cross-resistent in *in vivo* experimental systems with mercaptopurine (MP) and particularly that the combination of MP and MMPR produced synergism in experimental systems provided a major therapeutic lead (Table 1) [14, 15, 16]. MMPR alone proved ineffective in remission induction in patients with acute leukemia whether or not they had received prior MP [17]. However, the combination of MP and MMPR has produced a 44% complete remission/adequate trial rate and a 24% overall complete remission rate (Table 1) [18]. This is superior to the historical control MP where the overall complete remission rate was 9%. However, it remains possible that MP at different doses and schedules retested in a modern setting of supportive care might do as well as MP + MMPR. While a comparative study of MP and MP + MMPR has been considered the advent of other therapeutic programs with greater remission induction capacity has precluded this. Numerous studies in experimental systems involving variations in dose ratio, drug schedules, and different purine nucleoside analogues have failed to provide leads as to improving the effect of the combination. Accordingly, studies of MP plus MMPR for remission induction in AML were discontinued.

Arabinosyl cytosine (ara-C) is an effective antileukemic agent in experimental systems (Table 4). The daily administration of ara-C to mice bearing L 1210 leu-

Table 4. *Combined therapy with Ara-C and alkylating agents in L 1210 mouse leukemia*

Agent (S)	Schedule	Dose (Fraction of LD_{10})	Response: Increase in life span (median)	Response: "Cure"
Ara-C	Daily	1	200%	0
	Every 3 hrs. × 8 every 4 days	1	450%	0
Nitrosourea (CCNU)	Single dose	1	200%	0
	Every 3 hrs. × 8 every 4 days	1	80%	0
Ara-C + CCNU	Every 3 hrs. × 8 every 4 days	0.5	900%	90%

Treatment started 48 hrs. before death of controls i. e. at time when animals have 6—7×10^8 cells.

Table 5. *Ara-C and cyclophosphamide in AML*

Agent (s)	Schedule — dose	Total entered	Complete remission No.	Complete remission %	Source and Ref.
Ara-C	Daily	8	1	13%	MDA
		98	16	16%	ALGB
Ara-C	5 day courses of continuous infusion	16	5	31%	MDA
	every 2 wks.	83	25	30%	SWCCSG
Cyclophosphamide	Daily or weekly			<10%	ALGB
Ara-C + Cyclophosphamide	4 days courses every 2 wks.	32	14	41%	MDA

kemia results in a 2-fold increase in median survival. Ara-C inhibits DNA synthesis and affects only proliferating cells during the S-phase of the mitotic cycle. Since the generation time of L 1210 cells is 12 hours, intensive treatment through 1 or 2 cycles might prove more effective. This hypothesis was tested and, at the same cost in toxicity, intensive treatment over a 24-hour period every 4 days produced more than twice the antileukemic effect of daily treatment (Table 4) [19]. Thus, treatment designed to exploit knowledge of the cell kinetics of the tumor provided a therapeutic advantage. The generation time of acute myelogenous leukemia cells in man is 3 to 4 days [20]. Thus, treatment would have to be given for at least 4 days continuously in order to provide exposure of all of the proliferating cells to ara-C during the S period. Clinical studies relating to the use of ara-C in adults with AML are presented in Table 5. We discontinued our studies after 8 patients had been entered on daily ara-C when other experience as well as our own suggested that the complete remission rate was less than 20% [21, 22]. A pilot study was initiated wherein ara-C was given by continuous infusion over a 5-day period and such courses were repeated every 2 weeks. Five of 16 patients (31%) entered complete remission and in a more definitive study performed by the SWCCSG 30% of patients entered complete remission [23]. Thus, as in experimental systems, intermittent courses of treatment designed to cover at least one generation time of the neoplastic cells would appear to be superior to daily continuous treatment.

Several studies have indicated that the combination of an alkylating agent with ara-C is synergistic [24, 25]. One such study is illustrated in Table 4 period CCNU (a nitrosourea derivative) is an alkylating agent which alone is approximately as active as ara-C in the treatment of L 1210. When the two agents are combined, in a treatment program that produces toxicity comparable to the agents given alone, marked synergism is apparent. Thus, the combination produces a substantial 30-day survival ("cure") rate in contrast to the individual agents and for those animals dying of leukemia there is a marked increase in median life-span. The same observation holds when cyclophosphamide is substituted for CCNU. Since cyclophosphamide would appear to be somewhat superior to the nitrosoureas in the treatment of acute myelogenous leukemia, and is easier to manage in terms of host affects, it was employed in combination with ara-C in the clinical studies. The proportion of patients having adequate trials on the two drugs was approximately the same, and the overall complete remission rate was 41% for cyclophosphamide plus ara-C as compared to 31% for ara-C alone. The importance of the experimental observations and the suggested difference in these pilot studies have prompted a large multi-institute comparative study of ara-C and ara-C + cyclophosphamide. Thus, the relative efficacy of these programs should be known in the near future.

The efficacy of vincristine and prednisone in acute myelogenous leukemia has been controversial. However, remission rates as high as 20% have been observed with prednisone alone and recently vincristine has been found to produce objective remissions in the acute phase of chronic myelogenous leukemia [26, 27]. Moreover, prednisone and/or vincristine have produced an additive and perhaps synergistic increase in the response rate in patients with acute lymphocytic leukemia [5]. Prednisone and vincristine do not suppress the bone marrow. Because of this, it was possible, in preliminary studies, to add prednisone and vincristine to the ara-C plus cyclophosphamide program and not produce a significant increase of serious toxicity (Table 1 and 3). The resulting program (COAP) has produced an overall complete remission rate of 53%, and a complete remission/adequate trial rate of 71%. This study is continuing.

Discussion

The above is a summary of our attempts to improve the complete remission rate in adults with acute myelogenous leukemia. Prior to the early 1960's complete remission rates of, at most, 10% were achieved. With the introduction, particularly of Ara-C and daunomycin and of new techniques of combination and dose schedule manipulations, the complete remission rate has progressively improved so that with the last program (COAP) complete remissions have been achieved in the majority of patients (Table 2). It is important to emphasize that the median age of this group of patients is 55 years. The development of programs capable of producing complete remissions in the majority of patients is of major importance in view of the fact that, in acute lymphocytic leukemia and in Hodgkin's disease, this development served as a prelude to effective and quantitative studies of combined, cyclic, intensive, and dose-schedule studies during complete remission and thus a major prolongation of effective survival. It is hoped that this will prove possible in acute myelocytic leukemia.

It must be emphasized that advances in the effectiveness of chemotherapy programs have occurred *pari pasu* with advances in the supportive care of this disease. It is frequently difficult to unravel the relative contributions of supportive care and chemotherapy to the overall improvement in the complete remission rate. A simple and relatively accurate technique for doing this is to consider that the effectiveness of supportive care is a function of the fraction of patients achieving an adequate trial (provided patient selection is not skewed and the bone marrow toxicity of the treatment program is not excessive). The effectiveness of the chemotherapeutic program is a function of the complete remission rate over the number of patients having an adequate trial. A measure of the effectiveness of total treatment (chemotherapeutic + supportive care) is the complete remission rate for all the patients.

Summary

The rationale and the application of various chemotherapeutic programs to the treatment of acute myelogenous leukemia is reviewed. This includes the combination of MP and methylmercaptopurine riboside (MMPR); Ara-C; Ara-C combined with cyclophosphamide; and cyclophosphamide, vincristine, Ara-C and prednisone combination. The chemotherapeutic results are analyzed with respect to the proportion of patients achieving an adequate trial which is a measure primarily of the adequacy of supportive care. There has been progressive improvement in supportive care as evidenced by the fact that only 45% of patients treated with MP between 1958 and 1960 had an adequate trial as compared to 80% in the last two years. The complete remission rate for all patients has increaced from 10% for the MP group up to 53% for the 4 drug combined program. Preliminary results would indicate that the best dose schedule for Ara-C is 5 days of continuous infusion every two weeks.

References

1. FARBER, S., DIAMOND, L. K., MERCER, R. D., SYLVESTER, R. F., WOLFF, V. A.: Temporary remissions in acute leukemia in children produced by folic antagonist amethopteroylglutamic acid (aminopterin). New Engl. J. Med. **238**, 787—793 (1948).
2. BURCHENAL, J. H., MURPHY, M. L., ELLISON, R. R., SYKES, M. P., TAN, T. C., LEOME, L. A., KARNOFSKY, D. A., CRAVER, L. F., DARGEON, H. W., RHOADS, C. P.: Clinical evaluation of a new antimetabolite, 6-mercaptopurine in the treatment of leukemia and allied diseases. Blood **8**, 965—999 (1953).
3. SODEE, D. B., RUNDLES, R. W., SCHROEDER, L. R., HOOGSTRATEN, B., WOLMAN, I. J., TRAGGIS, D. G., COOPER, T., GENDEL, B. R., EBAUGH, F., TAYLOR, R.: Studies of sequential and combination antimetabolite therapy of acute leukemia: 6-mercaptopurine and methotrexate. Blood **18**, 431—454 (1961).
4. FREIREICH, E. J., KARON, M., FREI, E., III: Combined chemotherapy (VAMP) in the treatment of acute leukemia in children. Proc. Amer. Ass. Cancer Res. **5**, 20 (1964).
5. FREI, E., III, FREIREICH, E. M.: Progress and perspectives in the chemotherapy of acute leukemia. In: Advances in Chemotherapy, Vol. 2. New York: Academic Press Inc., p. 269.
6. SELAWRY, O.: Acute leukemia group B. New treatment schedule with improved survival in childhood leukemia. Intermittent parenteral versus daily oral administration of methotrexate for maintenance of induced remission. J. Amer. med. Ass. **194** (1), 75 (1965).

7. CHEVALIER, L., GLIDEWELL, O.: Schedule of mercaptopurine and effect of inducer drugs in prolongation of remission maintenance of acute leukemia. Proc. Amer. Ass. Cancer Res. **8**, 10 (1967).
8. ZUELZER, W. W.: Implications of long-term survival in acute stem cell leukemia of childhood treated with composite cyclic therapy. Blood **24**, 477—494 (1964).
9. HANANIAN, J., HOLLAND, J. F., SHEEHE, P.: Intensive chemotherapy of acute lymphocytic leukemia in children. Proc. Amer. Ass. Cancer Res. **6**, 26 (1965).
10. SKIPPER, H. E., SCHABEL, F. M., WILCOX, W. S.: Experimental evaluation of potential anticancer agents: XIII. On the criteria and kinetics associated with "curability" of experimental leukemia. Cancer Res. Rep. **35**, 111 (1964).
11. BURKITT, D., HUTT, M. S. R., WRIGHT, D. H.: The African lymphoma: preliminary observations on response to therapy. Cancer **18**, 399—410 (1965).
12. HERTZ, R., BERGENSTAL, D. M., LIPSETT, M. B., PRICE, E. B., HILBISH, T. F.: Chemotherapy of choriocarcinoma and related trophoblastic tumors in women. J. Amer. med. Ass. **168**, 845—855 (1958).
13. FREI, E., III: Studies of sequential and combination antimetabolite therapy of acute leukemia: 6-mercaptopurine and methotrexate. Blood **18**, 431 (1961).
14. BENNETT, L. L., JR., et al.: Activity and mechanism of action of 6-methylthiopurine ribonucleoside in cancer cells resistent to 6-mercaptopurine. Nature (Lond.) **205**, 1276—1279 (1965).
15. WANG, M. C., SIMPSON, A. I., PATERSON, A. R. P.: Combinations of 6-mercaptopurine and 6-methylmercaptopurine ribonucleoside in therapy of Ehrlich ascites carcinoma. Cancer Chemother. Rep. **51**, 101 (1967).
16. SCHABEL, F. M., LASTER, W. R., SKIPPER, H. E.: Chemotherapy of leukemia L1210 by 6-mercaptopurine in combination with 6-methylthiopurine ribonucleoside. Cancer Chemother. Rep. **51**, 111 (1967).
17. LUCE, J. K.: Clinical studies of 6-methylmercaptopurine riboside in acute leukemia. Cancer Chemother. Rep. **51**, 535 (1967).
18. BODEY, G. P.: Studies of combination 6-mercaptopurine and 6-methylmercaptopurine riboside in patients with acute leukemia and metastatic cancer. Cancer Chemother. Rep. **52**, 315 (1958).
19. SKIPPER, H. E., SCHABEL, F. M., WILCOX, W. S.: Experimental evaluation of potential anticancer agents: XXI. Scheduling of arabinosylcytosine to take advantage of its S-phase specificity against leukemic cells. Cancer Chemother. Rep. **51**, 125 (1967).
20. CLARKSON, B. T., OHKITA, R. T., OTA, K., FRIED, J.: Studies of cellular proliferation in human leukemia. I. Estimation of growth rates of leukemic and normal hematopoietic cells in 2 adults with acute leukemia given a single injection of tritiated thymidine. J. clin. Invest. **46**, 506 (1967).
21. ELLISON, R. R., HOLLAND, J. F.: Arabinosyl cytosine. A useful agent in the treatment of acute leukemia in adults. Blood **32**, 507 (1968).
22. BODEY, G. P., FREIREICH, E. J., MONTO, R. W., HEWLETT, J. S.: Cytosine arabinoside (NSC-63878) therapy for acute leukemia in adults. Cancer Chemother. Rep. **53**, 59—66 (169).
23. BICKERS, J., FREIREICH, E. J.: Personal communication.
24. EVANS, J. S., BOSTWICK, L., MENGEL, G. D.: Synergism of antineoplastic activity of cytosine arabinoside and perfiromycin. Biochem. Pharmacol. **13**, 983 (1964).
25. SCHABEL, F. M., JR.: In vivo leukemic cell kill kinetics and "curability" in experimental systems. In: The proliferation and spread of neoplastic cells. Baltimore: Williams and Wilkins Co. 1968, p. 379.
26. FREIREICH, E. J., GEHAN, E., FREI, E., III, SCHROEDER, L. R., WOLMAN, I. J., ANBARI, R., BARGERT, E. O., MILLS, S. D., PINKEL, D., SELAWRY, O. S., MOON, J. H., GENDEL, B. R., SPURR, C. L., STORRS, R., HAURANI, F., HOOGSTRATEN, B., LEE, S. (Acute leukemia group B): The effect of 6-mercaptopurine on the duration of steroid-induced remissions in acute leukemia: A model for evaluation of other potentially useful therapy. Blood **21**, 699—716 (1963).
27. CANELLOS, G. P., WHANG-PENG, J.: Effect of vincristine in blastic transformation of chronic granulocytic leukemia: Cytogenetic correlations. Abstract — Clin. Res., Vol. 1, No. 2. 1969, p. 402.

Induction of Remission in Acute Myeloid Leukemia

D. A. G. Galton

Institute of Cancer Research and Royal Postgraduate Medical School, London

The remission rate in acute myeloid leukaemia has undoubtedly increased in recent years mainly as a result of the introduction of more effective drugs, improvement in the techniques of using them, and of improvements in the supportive care of patients in a state of pancytopenia. Nevertheless, the results are unsatisfactory in comparison with those obtainable in the treatment of lymphoblastic leukaemia. To try to improve the results we must account for the difference.

I shall consider two of the many factors that determine the response to treatment; first the difference in sensitivity to cytotoxic drugs between the leukaemic blast cells and the normal haemopoietic cells, and secondly the capacity of the bone marrow to regenerate. We must first make the assumption, by no means established as correct, that in acute myeloid leukaemia as in lymphoblastic leukaemia, the leukaemic blast cells are genetically isolated from the normal bone-marrow stem cells from which they originated. In lymphoblastic leukaemia there is sufficient difference between the sensitivity to cytotoxic drugs of the leukaemic blast cells and the haemopoietic cells to make possible the destruction of many leukaemic blast cells relative to the number of haemopoietic cells. In acute myeloid leukaemia the difference in sensitivity is always less than in lymphoblastic leukaemia, but we may discern three groups of cases. In the first, the margin of difference, though small in comparison with what is found in lymphoblastic leukaemia is just sufficient to permit the differential destruction of blast cells with the survival of enough haemopoietic cells to regenerate normal bone marrow. These are the patients who remit. In the second group the difference in sensitivity to presently available cytotoxic drugs between the leukaemic blast cells and the haemopoietic cells is so slight that selective destruction is not possible. The treatment renders the bone marrow hypoplastic but leukaemic blast cells persist. Until we have more selective agents or until leucocyte transfusions or bone-marrow grafting become practicable we must accept an irreducible proportion of cases in which cytotoxic therapy will be ineffective and sometimes lethal.

The third group is important because it consists of patients who are potential remitters, but are easily harmed by chemotherapy. Their leukaemic blast cells are marginally more sensitive to cytotoxic drugs than their haemopoietic cells but the absolute number of residual haemopoietic cells is very small. The approach to cytotoxic therapy is thus of critical importance. Intensive therapy will be lethal if insufficient haemopoietic cells remain to repopulate the marrow however successfully the leukaemic blasts are eliminated. These are the patients who would be expected to benefit if the treatment were designed to induce remission in 2 stages. The first stage would be analogous to the initial treatment of lymphoblastic leukaemia with vincristine and prednisone in combination. Unfortunately this combination is not effective in acute myeloid leukaemia, and the only substitute is to use the myelosuppressive drugs at lower dosage or for shorter periods than would be used in the second stage, when the patient is in partial remission with more regenerating haemopoietic cells and less leukaemic blast cells in the bone marrow. The myelosuppressive drugs may now be used at higher dosage with less danger of inducing irreversible marrow hypoplasia. As the marrow regenerates and the number of blast cells continues to fall, the frequency of courses of treatment, and the size of the doses of the drugs employed could safely be increased to a level that would have led to the death of the patient if used as the first treatment.

The most intensive therapy therefore should be given when the patient is already going into remission, not when he is first treated. This approach might be expected to increase still further the overall remission rate and to reduce the proportion of fatalities resulting from treatment. In Great Britain the Medical Research Council's Working Party on Acute Leukaemia in Adults will shortly begin a comparative trial of three treatment schedules involving combinations of prednisone, mercaptopurine, cytosine arabinoside, daunorubicin and L-asparaginase. The schedules have been designed in accordance with the suggestion I have outlined, but the details are still being discussed and I cannot give the dose regimes that will be used.

The second factor that distinguishes the response to treatment of acute myeloid leukaemia from lymphoblastic leukaemia is the capacity of the bone marrow to regenerate after the leukaemic blast cells have been destroyed. In lymphoblastic leukaemia regeneration is characteristically rapid, and the new platelets, reticulocytes and neutrophils increase in numbers within a few days of each other. We are watching the normal response of a normal tissue under an intense stimulus to regenerate. A response of comparable speed and magnitude is rare in acute myeloid leukaemia. This failure cannot be due simply to the small numbers of residual haemopoietic stem cells because in many cases we see only partial regeneration in which the platelet count for example increases rapidly to normal but the reticulocyte and neutrophil counts remain low. In other cases regeneration proceeds slowly and incompletely, and the poor response is not clearly related either to the persistence of leukaemic blast cells or to the treatment administered.

Possible explanations are that the leukaemic blast cells are acting homeostatically to suppress the regeneration of the haemopoietic cells, or that the haemopoietic cells are abnormal and incapable of responding to normal regenerative stimuli. The latter explanation seems to fit the sequence of events in the poor response observed in many cases of myelomonocytic leukaemia. It is conceivable that in such cases, as in chronic granulocytic leukaemia, all the normal marrow stem cells have been replaced by a leukaemic clone. Clearly cytotoxic therapy could not be expected to succeed if this were true.

Summary

The induction of remission in acute leukaemia by cytotoxic drug therapy requires sufficient selectivity of cytotoxic action to achieve destruction of the leukaemic cells while ensuring the survival of sufficient haemopoietic stem cells to repopulate the bone marrow.

Sufficient selectivity exists frequently in lymphoblastic leukaemia but rarely in acute myeloid leukaemia. In the latter, the patient is most vulnerable at the start of treatment when the number of haemopoietic stem cells is very small in relation to the number of leukaemic blast cells. The incidence of remission might be increased by planning treatment in two stages. The drugs are first administered at moderate dosage to destroy sufficient leukaemic cells while permitting partial regeneration of haemopoietic cells; in the second stage, when the number of haemopoietic cells is larger in relation to the number of leukaemic blast cells, courses of treatment are administered more frequently and at higher dosage.

Complementary Chemotherapy in Acute Leukemia[1]

J. F. HOLLAND [2] and O. GLIDEWELL [3]

[2] Roswell Park Memorial Institute; New York State Department of Health; State University of New York at Buffalo; for the Acute Leukemia Group B

With 14 Figures

We shall interpret the term "complementary therapy" to include all forms of chemotherapy applied after remission induction. These include consolidation, intensification, maintenance therapy, and inducer dosing. We should like to define this latter term as the use of drugs ordinarily active for remission induction during the period when the patient is already in remission. In English the phrase "reinduction", which has also been used for this type of drug administration, is ambiguous. We now reserve that term for a second induction in individuals who have relapsed. Complementary therapy is probably not independent of the type treatment used for induction, although critical clinical experiments which bear on this point have not been reported.

The work we shall report has been performed over the last 13 years by the Acute Leukemia Group B which we have the privilege to serve as Chairman and Statistician.

Acute Myelocytic Leukemia

Evidence that complementary therapy is of importance in the types of disease called acute myelocytic leukemia is far more difficult to produce than for acute lymphocytic leukemia. In part, this may reflect the lesser effectiveness of remission induction agents which are available. In an early study in 1961 the ALGB studied remission duration in 125 patients with acute myelocytic leukemia induced into remission with 6-mercaptopurine. Only six patients reached complete remission status, and they were randomly allocated to 6-mercaptopurine or placebo. The study was abandoned because at the 5% response rate, it was concluded the study would require 800 patients and wouldn't finish till 1971; at the time of termination, how-

[1] These investigations were supported by Public Health Service Research Grants CA-2599 and CA-10456 from the National Cancer Institute, and by Grants to the principal investigators of the Acute Leukemia Group B: CA-03927-12, CA-04737-10, CA-14326-11, CA-05462-09, CA-11028-02, CA-04646-10, CA-03735-12, CA-04457-10, CA-07968-05, CA-08025-05, CA-05923-08, CA-07757-05 and CA-08080-05.

[2] Chairman.

[3] Statistician.

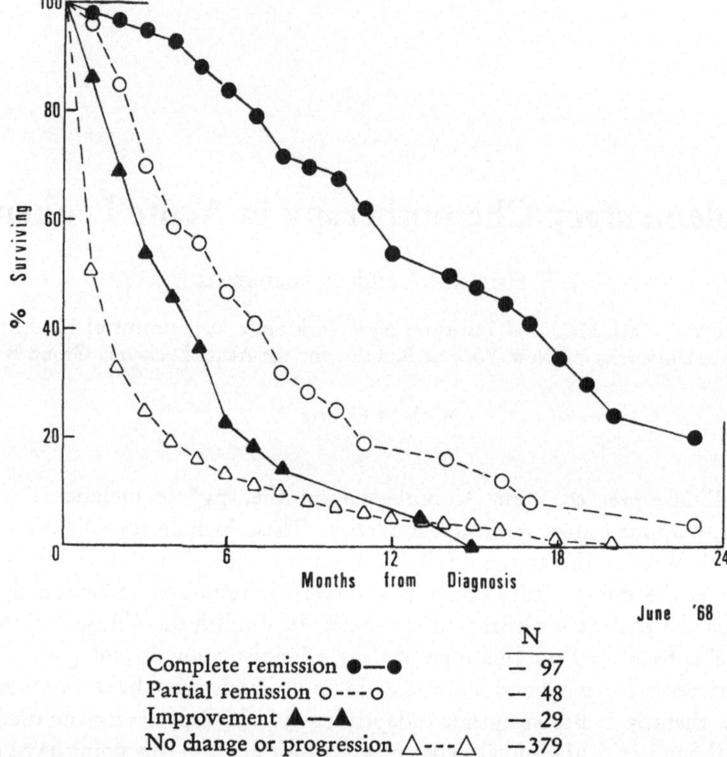

Fig. 1. Influence of chemotherapeutic response in acute myelocytic leukemia on survival

ever, the placebo maintained patients were faring somewhat better than those maintained on 6-MP [1].

With the advent of induction regimens which produce higher remission rates, we have approached the problem again. In Program 6513, a combination of vincristine, prednisone, 6-mercaptopurine and methotrexate was administered. After remission induction and repeated intensive courses of the drugs for consolidation, random allocation to further repetitive courses of complementary therapy or unmaintained remission was accomplished. The remission durations for both groups were virtually superimposable with a median of approximately five months [2].

Following extensive studies with daunorubicin for remission induction, median duration when maintained with cytosine arabinoside + methylglyoxal-bis-guanylhydrazone was 3 months, and for 6-mercaptopurine and methotrexate, four months [3].

One clearcut demonstration of effective complementary therapy in acute myelocytic leukemia has been the subcutaneous administration of cytosine arabinoside once weekly to patients induced into remission with that drug. The median duration of remission was 30 weeks compared to 5 weeks median for a randomly selected group who received no complementary treatment [4].

Although our data indicate longer median survival for those who enjoy complete remission (14 months) than partial remission (6 months), and those who enjoy only hematologic improvement (4 months) survive longer than individuals who fail to respond (1 month) (Fig. 1), we have not demonstrated that this is preponderantly due to complementary therapy [5]. We take it rather as an article of faith that when highly effective remission induction regimens are found, differences in complementary treatment regimens will also become more readily apparent. In large part, it is presumed that we are on the threshold of this discovery, since differences are emerging in induction regimens in acute myelocytic leukemia, whereas survival has not yet changed in these subtypes of acute leukemia. We are currently studying combinations of cytosine arabinoside with other drugs, and have preliminary evidence of sufficiently high remission induction and duration to presume that results soon to be tallied will change the pattern of complementary therapy in acute myelocytic leukemia.

In acute lymphocytic leukemia, the data are strikingly different. Early workers found that continuous treatment with folic acid antagonists appeared to be a more satisfactory therapeutic technique than deliberately allowing for relapse between successive remissions and then giving a repeat course. The first clear delineation of a maintenance activity independent of induction, however, was provided by FREIREICH and co-workers [6]. Previously untreated children, induced into remission with prednisone, were randomly allocated to 6-mercaptopurine or placebo for maintenance. A highly significant three-fold increase in remission duration was seen in those who received 6-mercaptopurine.

In a subsequent study, children who had relapsed from prior other treatments were induced with the combination of 6-mercaptopurine and prednisone, and then randomly allocated between 6-mercaptopurine maintenance and 6-mercaptopurine maintenance plus periodic vincristine and prednisone inducer doses [7]. The group receiving vincristine and prednisone inducer doses had considerably longer remissions. These data comprise the first proof that such inducer treatments exercise an effect on the leukemic population even though it was below the threshold of clinical detection. This observation constitutes a central concept in the advance in leukemia chemotherapy which has been made in recent years.

With the advent of daunorubicin, a third highly active agent for induction of remission in acute lymphocytic leukemia, we undertook another study of the same experimental design with 6-mercaptopurine [8]. Children relapsed from other treatments were induced with 6-mercaptopurine and prednisone and randomly allocated to one of four complementary therapy regimens: 6-mercaptopurine maintenance alone, 6-MP with inducer dosing of vincristine and prednisone, 6-MP with daunorubicin and prednisone, or 6-MP plus alternate vincristine and prednisone and daunorubicin and prednisone. The data have been decoded to the extent that the shortest remission is known to be ascribable to 6-mercaptopurine alone. The other three curves are still coded, but all represent prolongation of remission by use of the inducer agents. Since as yet there is no difference between the best two regimens, by coded subtraction one can calculate that at least one treatment involving prednisone and a single inducer drug must be as good as or better than the combination of the inducer drugs given alternately.

The classic experiments of GOLDIN et al. demonstrated no significant difference in median survival among methotrexate dose schedules in advanced leukemia L 1210, whereas superiority of intermittent methotrexate every 4th day at the higher doses which were thereby tolerable was readily apparent in early leukemia [9]. An attempt to validate this in man was undertaken. Methotrexate induction was allocated at

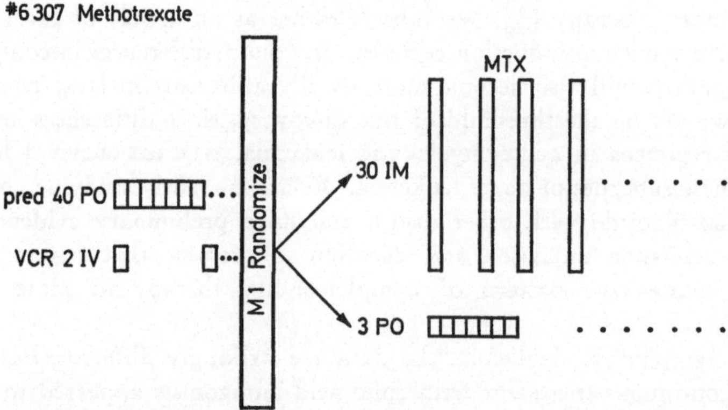

Fig. 2. Schema of induction and maintenance in study 6307 (11)

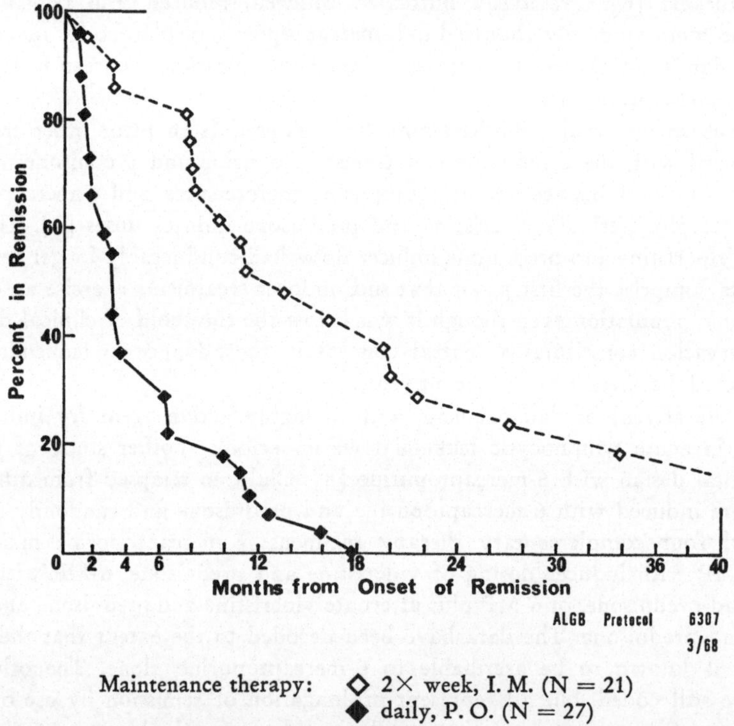

Maintenance therapy: ◇ 2× week, I. M. (N = 21)
◆ daily, P. O. (N = 27)

Fig. 3. Updated results of study 6307. Twice weekly parenteral methotrexate produces longer remissions than daily oral drug administration

random to daily or intermittent twice weekly schedule, followed by maintenance on daily or intermittent methotrexate after re-randomization. No difference was found in remission induction (31% and 28%), although the interrupted methotrexate schedule afforded longer remissions [10]. These observations were consistent with GOLDIN's findings. At that time, vincristine became available and the high activity of vincristine and prednisone in inducing remission was recognized. Thereafter, we

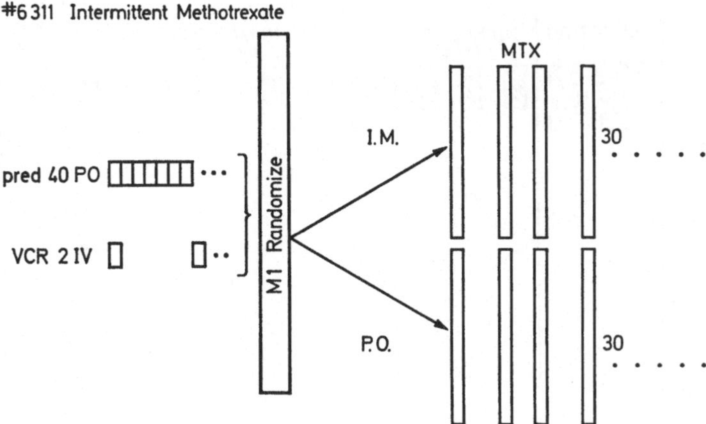

Fig. 4. Schema of induction and maintenance in study 6311 (12)

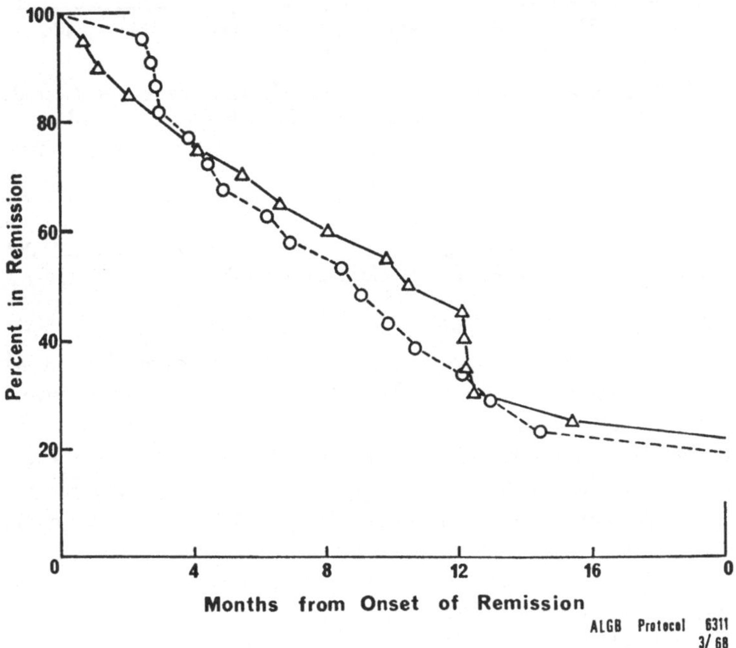

Maintenance therapy: ○ MTX, I. M. (22 cases)
△ MTX, P. O. (20 cases)

Fig. 5. Similarity of remission duration when treated with methotrexate given twice weekly either intramuscular (i. m.) or orally (p. o.) (12)

studied a group of children with no prior treatment who were induced into remission with vincristine and prednisone and then randomly allocated to oral daily methotrexate or parenteral twice weekly high dose drug (Fig. 2). A highly significant difference in remission duration favoring the twice weekly parenteral methotrexate over the oral daily dose developed (Fig. 3). This permitted the interpretation that either the schedule or the route might have been the important factor in producing

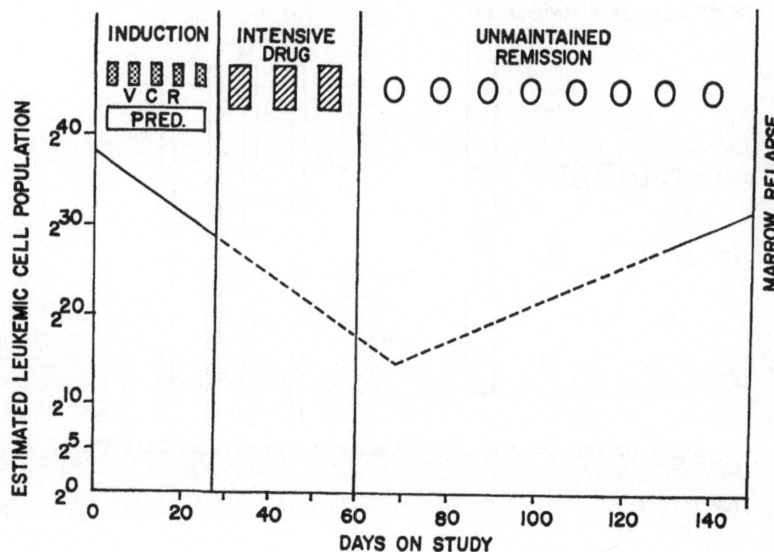

Fig. 6. Schematic representation of induction and consolidation treatment succeeded by unmaintained remission. The estimated leukemic cellular body burden is plotted against time to describe tumor behavior following treatment. Estimates have been made from percentage of leukemic cells in frequent marrow aspirations, estimates of cellularity, marrow size, hepatic and splenic size, node size and extent, and blood content of leukemic cells. The dashed lines represent extrapolations when marrow content of leukemic cells is so low it precludes identification and direct calculation — 2^{10} approximates 10^3, 2^{20} approximates 10^6, 2^{30} approximates 10^9, 2^{40} approximates 10^{12}

the improvement [11]. Accordingly, a study design was undertaken in which vincristine and prednisone induction was followed by methotrexate administration twice weekly either parenterally or orally at random (Fig. 4). No evidence of effect of route of administration was found [12] (Fig. 5). We are left with the proposition that administering methotrexate twice weekly produces substantially improved complementary therapy compared to the older conventional daily administration. In part, this is surely attributable to the higher dose which is administered in the interrupted schedule. The observation is also drug specific, however, insofar as interrupted high dose parenteral treatment with 6-mercaptopurine was not superior to its oral daily administration [7].

ALGB studies of cyclophosphamide maintenance and vincristine maintenance do not indicate that these drugs are among the most active compounds for this purpose [13, 14]. The Australian Cancer Society's Childhood Leukemia Study Group, however, has recently reported substantial activity of vincristine in remission maintenance of acute lymphocytic leukemia [15]. Induction was accomplished with prednisolone for five days and with weekly injections of vincristine. The median remission time was 10 to 12 months, and 21% of the children were maintained for over 2 years [16]. This observation tends to modify the concept of exclusive induction and maintenance drugs since vincristine appears to have evidence for both activities. In our own prior observations on vincristine as a maintenance agent, we concluded that there was insignificant maintenance activity [14]. The major difference between

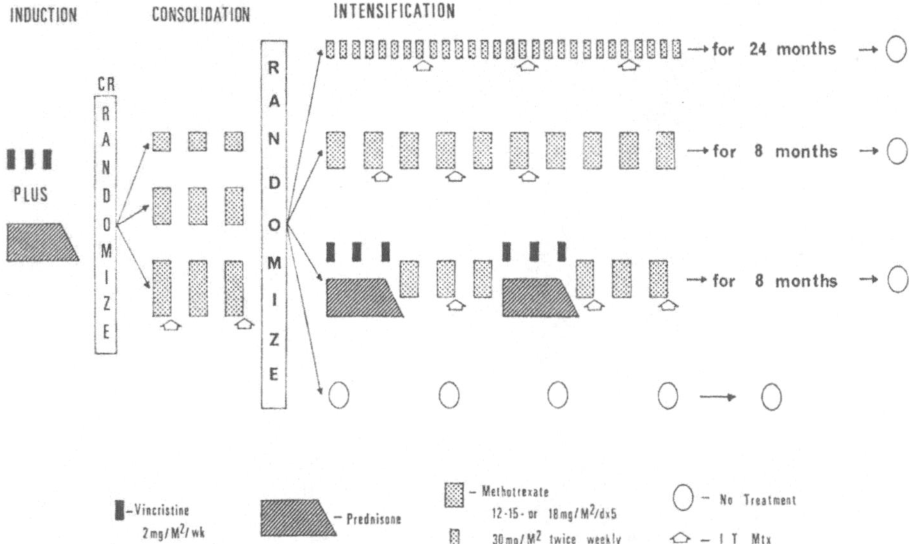

Fig. 7. Schema of induction, consolidation, intensification and induced dosing in study 6601

our earlier study and the recent Australian contribution is that only 5 of 117 evaluable patients in our program had had no prior treatment, whereas the Australian children had previously been untreated. The influence of changes in the host and the leukemia during progression of the disease thus affords major emphasis to the importance of the first therapy administered.

Perhaps the most significant alteration in the strategy of our complementary therapy has derived from the recognition that much fundamental information can be learned about the residual leukemic population by observing the time to relapse after cessation of treatment. This bioassay system has provided a gross appraisal of the leukemocidal effect of a treatment under study, by estimates of the residual leukemic cellular body burden. This has allowed succeeding experimental designs to optimize the best leukemocidal effects (Fig. 6). Thus, consolidation and intensification rather than maintenance treatment have dominated certain study designs for complementary therapy. These studies have been influenced strongly by the work of SKIPPER, SCHABEL and WILCOX [17]. When the unmaintained remission time after 3 intensive 5-day courses of methotrexate was found to be short, a calculation of residual leukemic body burden was made. This was based on the rate of disappearance of marrow leukemic infiltration and the rate of repopulation during subsequent relapse, with extrapolations of these two slopes to the nadir. The calculated residual leukemic cells were high and this was thought probably due to inadequate duration of the intensive treatment. Since 120 days calculated to be the time at which leukemocidal effect would be complete, if the killing rate was similar to that observed during early induction, we designed a program of consolidation and intensification treatment with repeated courses of methotrexate which deliberately lasted twice that long or 240 days (Fig. 7). For comparison purposes, there was again 3 courses only. In "Regimen D" of this study 6601, intermittent inducer doses of vincristine and prednisone were also given during the 8 months of courses. The data demonstrate that there is longer un-

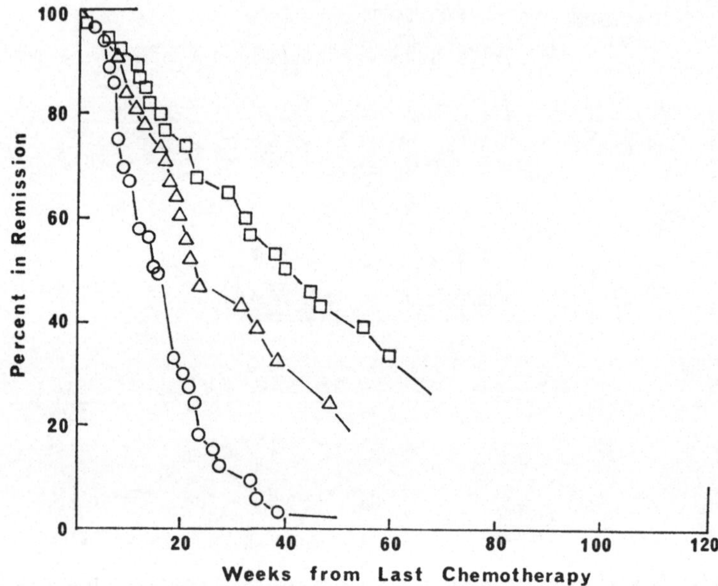

Fig. 8. Unmaintained remission durations of three regimes of Study 6601. See Fig. 7. ○ MTX 3 courses (N =36); △ MTX 8 months of courses (N = 34); □ MTX 8 months of courses plus inducers (N = 40)

maintained remission after 8 months of courses than after the 3 courses (Fig. 8). We interpret this to mean that during the 8 months of repeated intensive courses, more leukemic cells were found in the S phase of the cell cycle and were exposed to lethal effects of methotrexate, and hence the residual body burden was lower. In addition it is possible, although not proven, that the repopulating cells after 8 months of courses were so selected that the faster multiplying cell types had been eliminated leaving as lower growing leukemia. In "Regimen D", interspersed between each third course of methotrexate, 3 injections of vincristine and 2 weeks of prednisone were administered. The unmaintained remission time was substantially longer. This is another demonstration of the effect of inducer doses. Forty percent are still in unmaintained remission after 1 year. This is tacit evidence that human leukemic populations contain cells in G_0 or prolonged G_1 cell cycle phases. There is good basis to estimate the leukemic body burden of the child with florid leukemia as approximately 10^{11}—10^{12} cells [18]. Earlier conjectures that orderly geometric growth with a doubling time of 4 days was characteristic of leukemic cell kinetics must obviously be faulty in some respect.

We consider the interrelationships of drug, dose schedule, first treatment, induction, consolidation, intensification, maintenance, inducer drugs and complicating diseases and their treatment all to be relevant to remission duration and all to be influenced in part by the immunity of the host. In this respect, it is of interest to recognize the contribution that irradiated allogenic leukemic cell and/or BCG immunization has made to unmaintained remission time in the experiments of MATHÉ and co-workers [19]. These data are comparatively plotted with those for "Regimen D" of Protocol 6601 (where no exogenous immunogens were given) (Fig. 9).

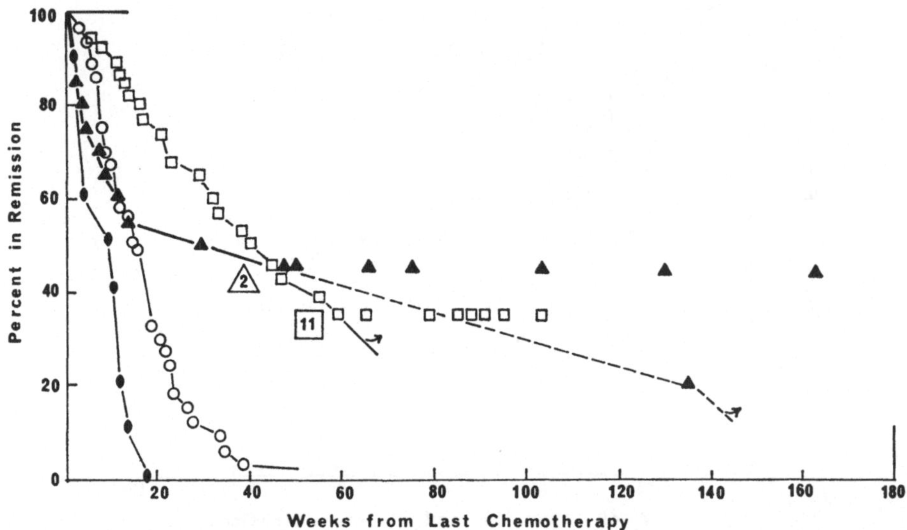

Fig. 9. Unmaintained remission time of patients treated by MATHÉ et al. (19) with immunotherapy after completion of chemotherapy, and in "Regimen D" of 6601, untreated after completion of drug administration. The projection of the life table estimate levels point to the worst possible results. The points not on lines are the patients still in unmaintained remission more than 1 year. The numbers in the triangle and square indicate the number of patients still in remission less than one year. ● MATHÉ; Controls (N = 10); ▲ MATHÉ; Immunotherapy (N = 20); ○ MTX 3 courses (N = 36); □ MTX 8 months of courses plus inducers (N = 40)

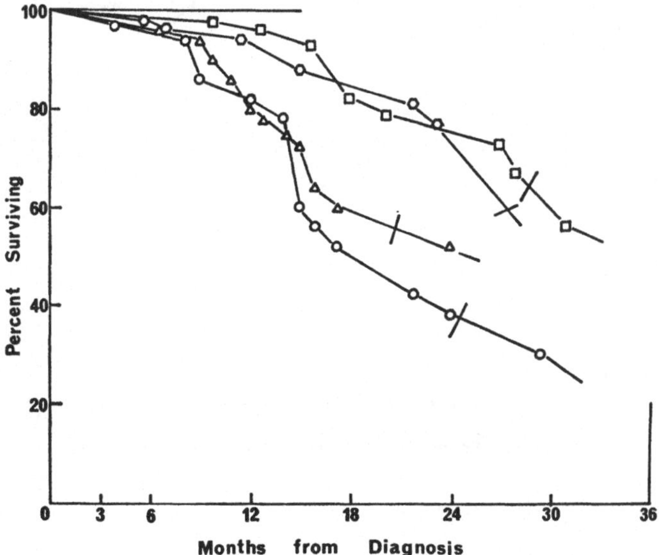

Fig. 10. Influence of first methotrexate treatment course (after vincristine and prednisone induction) on survival. ○ MTX 3 courses (N = 36); △ MTX 8 months of courses (N = 55); □ MTX 8 months of courses plus inducers (N = 54); ⬡ MTX 2× week (N = 57) / Fewer than 10 patients observed

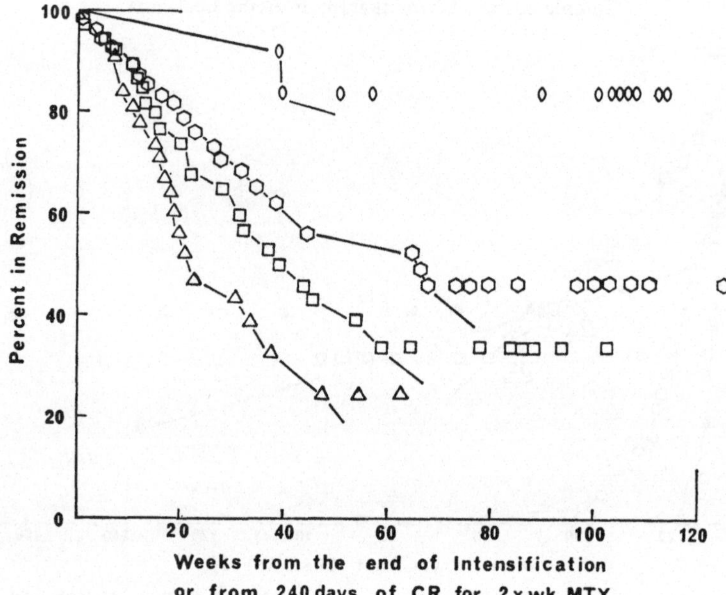

Fig. 11. Relapsing rates for several chemotherapy regimens plotted as unmaintained duration after 8 months of courses △ or after 8 months of courses plus vincristine and prednisone inducer dosing □. The comparable relapsing rate for patients receiving twice weekly methotrexate after three courses of the drug are shown ⬡. The effect of eight months of methotrexate (with or without vincristine plus prednisone inducer dosing) then followed by twice weekly methotrexate is shown. 0 2× week MTX after △ or □ (N = 14)

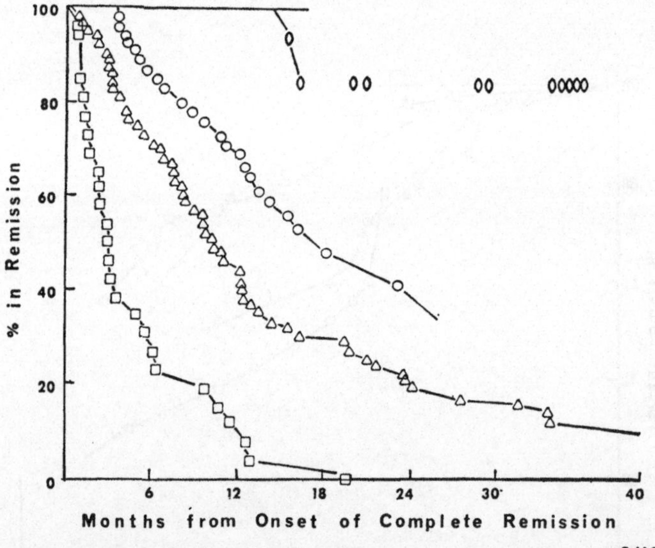

No methotrexate courses before maintenance. □, △
Three methotrexate courses. ○
Eight months of courses (some with vincristine and prednisone inducer dosing before maintenance). 0

Fig. 12. Comparison of maintenance regimes of methotrexate daily or twice weekly as influenced by intensity of prior methotrexate courses. All patients were entered into remission with vincristine and prednisone

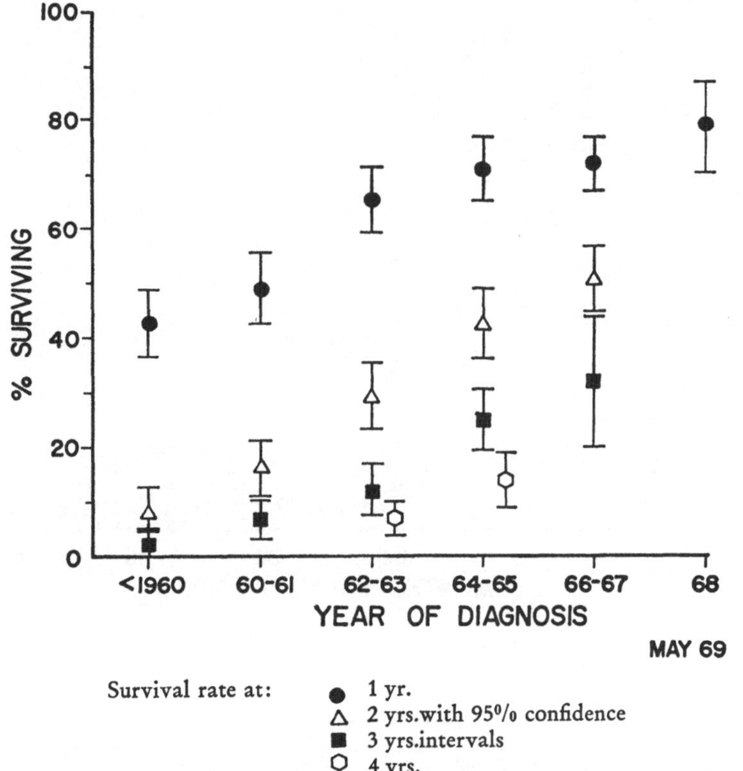

Survival rate at: ● 1 yr.
△ 2 yrs. with 95% confidence
■ 3 yrs. intervals
○ 4 yrs.

Fig. 13. Increasing percentages of children with acute leukemia are surviving longer periods. The data imply that increasing survivorship at 2, 3, and 4 years follows behind 1 year survivals and roughly parallels it. We can therefore anticipate a much higher proportion of 4 year survivors in 1968 than seen in 62—63

This comparison indicates that the results following immunotherapy are not uniquely long, but they do appear to represent a "break" in the curve. One must still speculate what the results of immunotherapy would be after a regimen of chemotherapy of the efficacy of "Regimen D".

In a further comparison of regimens in 6601, one can appreciate that those who received three courses of methotrexate only did not survive so long as those who received the 8 months of treatment, or particularly the 8 months with inducer dosing, or three courses and then two years of intermittent methotrexate (Fig. 10). Accordingly, one must consider very searchingly the design of studies in the future where substantial therapy bordering on maximal is not administered at the outset. It appears that a permanent impairment can follow inadequate early treatment, and despite other chemotherapeutic attempts, survival is compromised.

A further evidence of the importance of intensive treatment is seen in Fig. 11. The unmaintained remission times for Regimens C and D, 8 months of methotrexate courses, with inducer doses of vincristine and prednisone in D, are shown. The remission curve for Regimen B (3 courses of methotrexate and then twice weekly drug) is also shown, with the plot commencing at 8 months to make it comparable. The twice

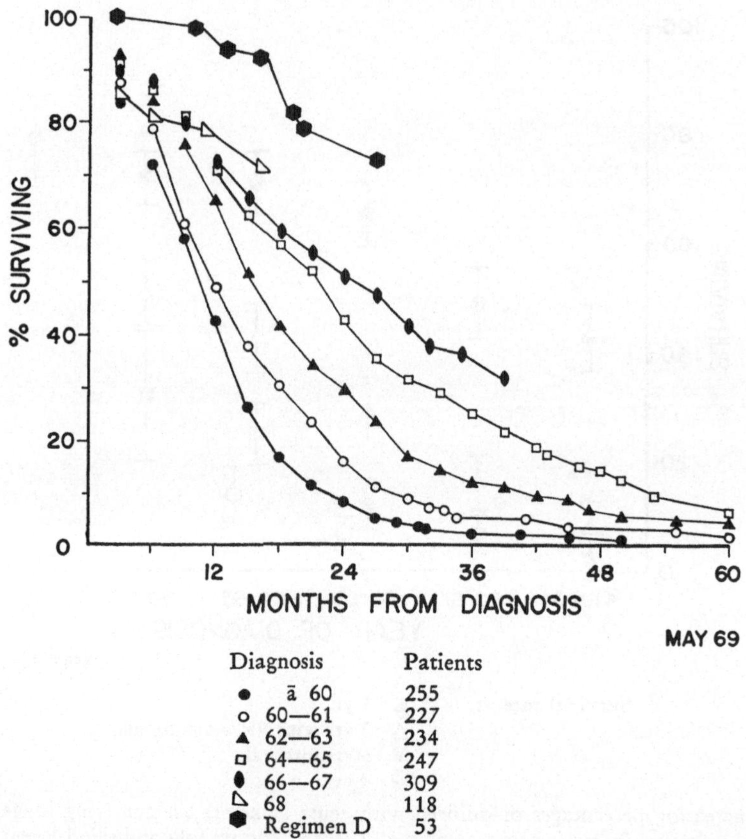

Fig. 14. Survival curves plotted by life table methods for all patients less than 20 years with acute lymphocytic leukemia who entered ALGB studies. Regimen D is also represented in the 66—67 curve. The projections of incomplete curves suggest that a large number of 5-year survivors will be observed. Among them may be individuals who will never relapse

weekly maintenance of B is somewhat better than the unmaintained responses of C and D. If, however, twice weekly maintenance treatment was initiated after the 8 months of courses in C and D, as it was in a small number before we changed the protocol, the remission duration is markedly enhanced, with approximately 80% still in remission at 80 weeks. This is the best complementary treatment on which we have data. The relationships to other techniques of using methotrexate in consolidation and maintenance is shown in Fig. 12.

Finally, in the course of the last decade, with the advent of new drugs, techniques, and a few glimmers of enlightenment, there has been progressive increase in survival of children with acute lymphocytic leukemia. Survivorship at 1, 2, and 3 and 4 years is increasing (Fig. 13). This is not all ascribable to the improvements in general medical care since similar observations have not been made in all clinics or in all collaborating groups of investigators.

In the last figure survival experiences are plotted in a different and more conventional manner in order to show the data for "Regimen D" of 6601 (Fig. 14). It must be recalled that the initial chemotherapy in these children was terminated after

8 months of methotrexate courses with vincristine plus prednisone inducer dosing. More intensive and prolonged treatment might well provide a further step toward eradication of the disease. Such studies are in progress.

Summary

Complementary therapy, that chemotherapy administered after induction of remission, has been generally inactive in patients with acute myelocytic leukemia. Cytosine arabinoside is the first drug in the experience of the Acute Leukemia Group B to show evidence of maintenance activity.

In acute lymphocytic leukemia, twice weekly methotrexate is superior to daily drug administration. Repeated intensive 5-day courses of methotrexate cause prolonged unmaintained remission. When vincristine and prednisone are interspersed with the methotrexate courses, given over 8 months, subsequent unmaintained remission exceeds one year in 40%, which is equeal to the data reported for immunotherapy. When the intensive courses of methotrexate are followed by twice weekly methotrexate maintenance, remission duration is the longest we have observed.

The survival of patients with acute lymphocytic leukemia is improving, with predictable proportions reaching 5 years without relapse.

References

1. Lee, S.: ALGB minutes. 6-MP remission study report. Nov. 26, 1961. Unpublished observations.
2. Henderson, E. C.: ALGB minutes. Protocol 6513/A. July 14, 1967. Unpublished observations.
3. Bernard, J. Boiron, M., Weil, M., Jacquillat, C.: ALGB minutes. Protocols 6706 and 6706 A Sept. 7, 1968. Unpublished observations.
4. Ellison, R. R., Holland, J. F., Weil, M., Jacquillat, C., Boiron, M., Bernard, J., Sawitsky, A., Rosner, F., Gussoff, B., Silver, R. T., Karanas, A., Cuttner, J., Spurr, C. L., Hayes, D. M., Blom, J., Leone, A. A.: Arabinosyl cytosine: a useful agent in the treatment of acute leukemia in adults. Blood **32**, 507—523 (1968).
5. — Glidewell, O. J., Holland, J. F.: Prognostication of survival of adults with acute myelocytic leukemia (AML). Proc. Amer. Ass. Cancer Res. **10**, 22 (1969).
6. Freireich, E. J., Gehan, E., Frei, E. III, Schroeder, L. R., Wolman, I. J., Anbari, R., Burgert, E. O., Mills, S. D., Pinkel, D., Selawry, O. S., Moon, J. H., Gendel, B. R., Spurr, C. L., Storrs, R., Haurani, F., Hoogstraten, B., Lee, S.: The effect of 6-mercaptopurine on the duration of steroid-induced remissions in acute leukemia: a model for evaluation of other potentially useful therapy. Blood **21**, 699—716 (1963).
7. Chevalier, L., Glidewell, O.: Schedule of 6-MP and effect of inducer drugs on remission maintenance in acute leukemia. Proc. Amer. Ass. Cancer Res. **8**, 10 (1967).
8. Kung, F.: ALGB minutes, protocol 6608. March 1969. Unpublished observations.
9. Goldin, A., Venditti, J. M., Humphreys, S. R., Mantel, N.: Modification of treatment schedules in the management of advanced mouse leukemia with amethopterin. J. nat. Cancer Inst. **17**, 203—212 (1956).
10. Selawry, O. S., James, D.: Therapeutic index of methotrexate as related to dose schedule and route of administration in children with acute lymphocytic leukemia. Proc. Amer. Ass. Cancer Res. **6**, 54 (1965).
11. — Hananian, J., Wolman, I. J., Abir, E., Chevalier, L., Gourdeau, R., Denton, R., Gussoff, B. D., Levy, R., Burgert, O., Jr., Mills, S. D., Blom, J., Jones, B., Patterson, R. B., McIntyre, O. R., Haurani, F. I., Moon, J. H., Hoogstraten, B., Kung, F. Y., Sheehe, P. R., Frei, E. III, Holland, J. F.: New treatment schedule with improved survival in childhood leukemia. J. Amer. med. Ass. **194**, 75—81 (1965).
12. Acute leukemia group B: acute lymphocytic leukemia in children. Maintenance therapy with methotrexate administered intermittently. J. Amer. med. Ass. 207, 923—928 (1969).

13. HOOGSTRATEN, B., SCHROEDER, L. R., FREIREICH, E. J., FREI, E. III, HOLLAND, J., PINKEL, D., VOGEL, P., MILLS, S. D., BURGERT, E. O., JR., HAYES, D. M., SPURR, C. L., KURKCUOGLU, M., STORRS, R., EBAUGH, F., WOLMAN, I. J., HAURANI, F., GENDEL, B., GEHAN, D.: Cyclophosphamide (cytoxan) in acute leukemia, preliminary report. Cancer Chemother. Rep. **8**, 116—119 (1960).
14. KARON, M., FREIREICH, E. J., FREI, E. III, TAYLOR, R., WOLMAN, I. J., DJERASSI, I., LEE, S, L., SAWITSKY, A., HANANIAN, J., SELAWRY, O., JAMES, D., JR., GEORGE, P., PATTERSON, R. B., BURGERT, O., JR., HAURANI, F. I., OBERFIELD, R. A., MACY, C. T., HOOGSTRATEN, B., BLOM, J.: The role of vincristine in the treatment of childhood acute leukemia. Clin. Pharmacol. Ther. **7**, 332—339 (1966).
15. Australian Cancer Society's Childhood Leukaemia Study Group: Cyclic drug regimen for acute childhood leukemia. Lancet **1968 I**, 313—319.
16. COLEBATCH, J. H., BAIKIE, A. G., CLARK, A. C. L., JONES, D. L., LEE, C. W. G., LEWIS, I. C., NEWMAN, N. M.: Cyclic regimen for childhood leukemia. Lancet **1968 II**, 869.
17. SKIPPER, H. E., SCHABEL, F. M., JR., WILCOX, W. S.: Experimental evaluation of potential anticancer agents. XIII. On the criteria and kinetics associated with "curability" of experimental leukemia. Cancer Chemother. Rep. **35**, 3—111 (1964).
18. HOLLAND, J. F.: Clinical studies of unmaintained remissions in acute lymphocytic leukemia. In: The proliferation and spread of neoplastic cells.
19. MATHÉ, G., AMIEL, J. L., SCHWARZENBERG, L., SCHNEIDER, M., CATTAN, A., SCHLUMBERGER, J. R., HAYAT, M., DE VASSAL, F.: Active immunotherapy for acute lymphoblastic leukemia. Lancet **1969 I**, 697—699.

Methods and Strategy for the Treatment[1] of Acute Lymphoblastic Leukemia

G. MATHÉ, J. L. AMIEL, L. SCHWARZENBERG, M. SCHNEIDER, A, CATTAN, M. HAYAT, F. DE VASSAL, and J. R. SCHLUMBERGER

Institut de Cancérologie et d'Immunogénétique Hôpital Paul-Brousse, 14 Avenue Paul-Vaillant-Couturier, 94-Villejuif, France, and Institut Gustave Roussy, 16 bis, Avenue Paul-Vaillant-Couturier, 94-Villejuif, France

With 19 Figures

Acute lymphoblastic leukaemia (A. L. L.) is a malignant disease in which the proliferating cells are conventionally identified as "lymphoblasts", cells that are theoretically the precursors of lymphocytes (see MATHÉ and SÉman, 1963).

As a general rule, this proliferation begins and is predominant in the bone marrow and, broadly speaking, has two main types of effect: the signs and symptoms that arise as a direct consequence of the leukaemic cells in the tissues (bone pain, lymphadenopathy, splenomegaly, hepatomegaly, leukaemic meningitis, testicular enlargement ...); other signs are an indirect consequence of the leukaemic proliferation being, in the main, myeloid insufficiency (anaemia, neutropenia, thrombocytopenia and their consequences, tiredness, infection and haemorrhage).

Fundamental treatment is to attempt to inhibit the leukaemic cell population; the consequences of myeloid insufficiency are treated symptomatically. In this review, we shall be particularly concerned with the treatment of leukaemic cell proliferation.

In the virus-induced leukaemias of chickens, mice and cats, the appearance of the virus particles, as revealed by electron microscopy is the same for all species. SÉMAN (1968, 1968), working in our laboratory has observed similar particles in human leukaemia but, so far, no bio-assay has been devised to prove that these viruses have, in fact, caused human leukaemia. Nevertheless, it is not unreasonable, at the present time, to try methods of therapy that are directed against this probable viral factor.

We will describe successively, the methods of therapy that are available, the strategy by which they can be used in combination, in the light of their mechanisms and modes of action, with a view to try to cure the patient; finally, we shall consider symptomatic treatment.

---

[1] This work was carried out with the acid of I.N.S.E.R.M., contract no. 66-235 and D.G.R.S.T. contract no. 68.01.134.

I. Methods

1. *Chemotherapy* is the principal method for the treatment of acute leukaemia; since FARBER and his colleagues (1948) demonstrated, twenty years ago, that aminopterin enabled apparently complete regressions to be obtained, there has been an increase in the number and types of drugs that, with varying efficiency, can be used to induce remissions, but their effect is only to induce a remission for, in every case, this has been followed by a relapse.

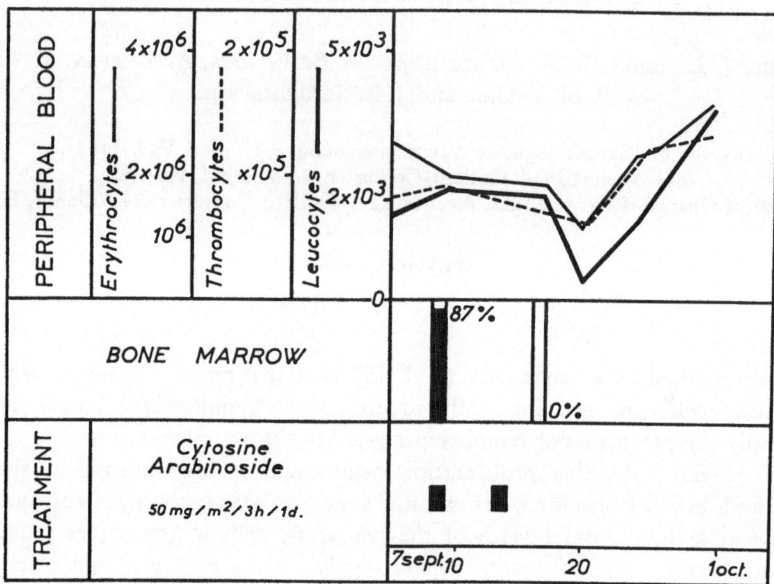

Fig. 1. Induction of a remission in a patient suffering from acute lymphoblastic leukaemia with cytosine arabinoside, given according to the method proposed by SKIPPER for the treatment of L 1210 leukaemia in mice

Table 1 lists the more widely used drugs in each pharmalogical group and the frequency of apparently complete remissions that they can induce in various therapeutic regimes. The percentages in this Table are not strictly comparable, the proportion of children in relation to adults, and the proportion of first visible phases of the disease [2] in relation to relapse were variable; the frequency of remissions is higher in children than in adults and remission is more frequently induced in the first visible phase than in relapse. The definition of an "apparently complete remission" varies from one author to another.

Fig. 1 to 7 give examples of remissions we have obtained either using drugs that have been available for a long time, though their method of administration is recent, (cytosine arabinoside, 50 mg/m²/3 h for 24 hours once a week; methotrexate, 75 mg/m²/8 h for 48 hours followed by folinic acid), or using new drugs (dauno-

[2] The patient is said to be "in a visible phase" of the disease when it gives rise to one or more signs and symptoms. When the manifestations of leukaemia can no longer be detected, the disease is in an "apparently complete remission".

Table 1. *Value of various compounds to induce remissions in acute lymphoblastic leukaemia*

Groups of compounds	Compounds	Modalities of administration	Frequency of complete remission	References
Steroids	Prednisone	1 mg/kg/d	57%	Freireich, Gehan et al., 1963
		3 mg/kg/d	74%	Bernard, Weil et al., 1962
		100 mg/m²/d	58%	Mathé, Schwarzenberg et al., 1966
Antipurines	6-mercpatopurine	90 mg/m²/d	27%	Frei et al., 1961 Burchenal et al., 1963
Antifolics	Methotrexate	3 mg/m²/d	21%	Frei et al., 1961
		30 mg/m²/d	31%	Selawry and James, 1965
		MTX: 75 mg/m²/8h×6 F. Ac.: 25 mg/m²/6h×16	40%	Mathé et al., 1969
Antipyrimidines	Cytosine arabinoside	100 mg/m²/d	20 to 50%	Henderson and Burke, 1965 Yu and Clarkson, 1966 Bernard, Boiron et al., 1966
		50 mg/m²/3h×8 weekly	17%	Schwarzenberg et al., 1969
Alkylating agents	Cyclophosphamide	100 mg/m²/d	8 to 18%	Mathé, Schweisguth, Brulé et al., 1963 Fernbach et al., 1962 Tan et al., 1961
	B.C.N.U.	150 mg/m²/d/×3	13%	Pers. exp. (not publish.)
	Methyl-glyoxal bis (G—H)	150 to 200 mg/m²/2 d	12%	Schwarzenberg, Schneider et al., 1966
	I.C.R.F. 159	7 to 109 mg/kg/d	0/9	Hellmann et al., 1969
		300 mg/m²/d	2/7	Mathé et al., 1969
Alkaloid of catharanta rosea	Vincristine	1 mg/m²/weekly	43%	Mathé, Schweisguth, Brulé, Brézin et al., 1963
Extracts of streptomyces ceruleo-rubidus	Rubidomycin	10 to 20 mg/m²/3 d	22%	Mathé, Amiel, Hayat et al., 1967 [a]
			60%	Jacquillat, Najean et al., 1967
			25%	OERTC (leukaemia group) (not publ.)
Extract of streptomyces peucetius caesius	Adriamycin	10 to 15 mg/m²	1/5	Bonadonna et al., 1969
			≠ id.	Mathé et al. (not published)
Extract of E. coli	L-asparaginase	10 to 200 U/kg/d	11/21 [b]	Hill et al., 1968
			36%	Burchenal, Karnofsky, Murphy and Oettgen, 1968
		35.000 U/m²/d	39%	Mathé, Amiel et al., 1969

[a] Original publication; the percentage of remissions may not correspond, they had been brought up to date. [b] "Marked and rapid response".

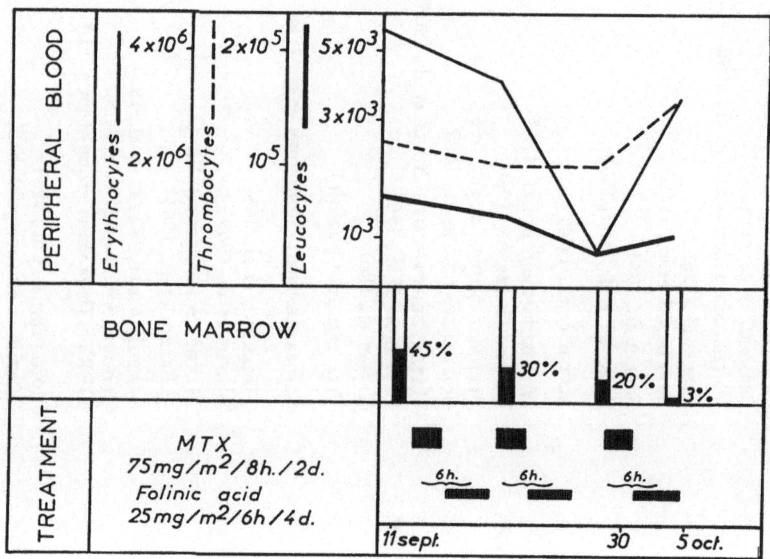

Fig. 2. Induction of a remission in a patient suffering from acute lymphoblastic leukaemia with the combination of methotrexate and folinic acid

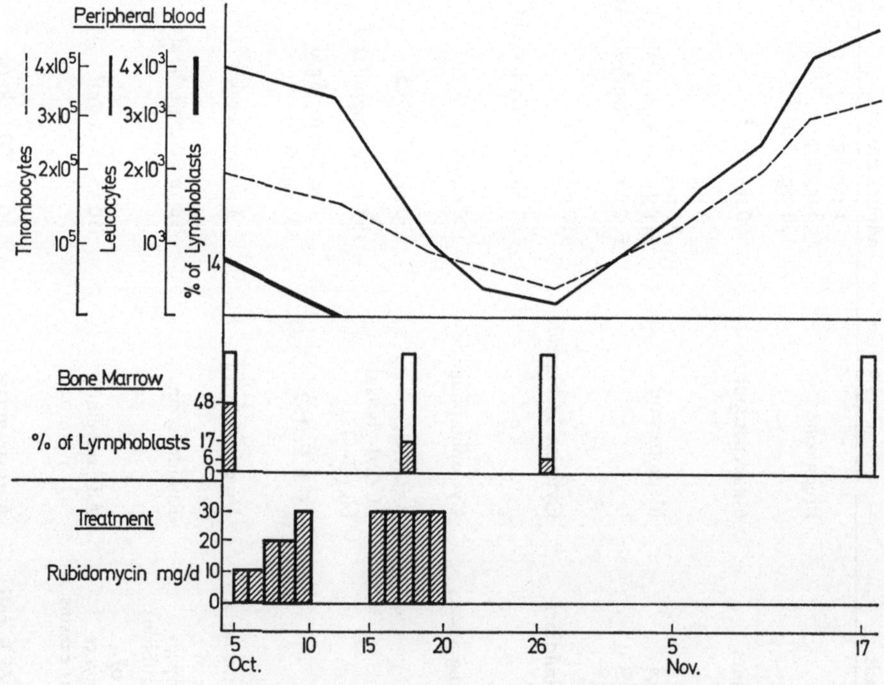

Fig. 3. Induction of a remission with daunomycin in an acute lymphoblastic leukaemic patient

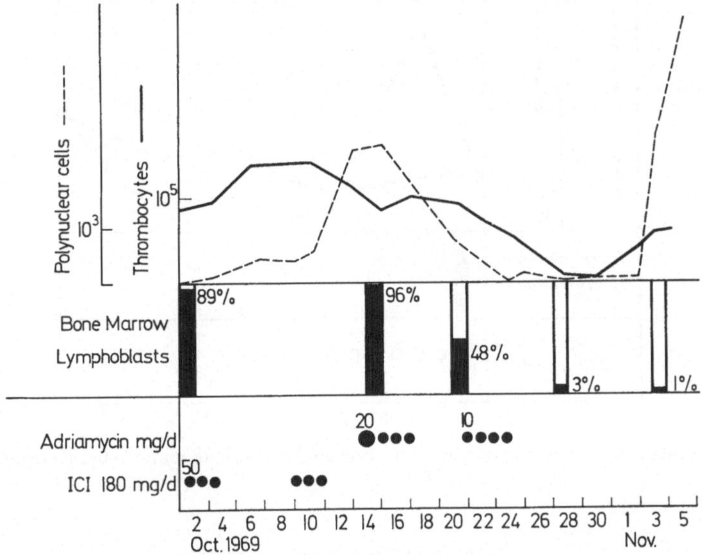

Fig. 4. Induction of a remission in a patient suffering from acute lymphoblastic leukaemia with adriamycin

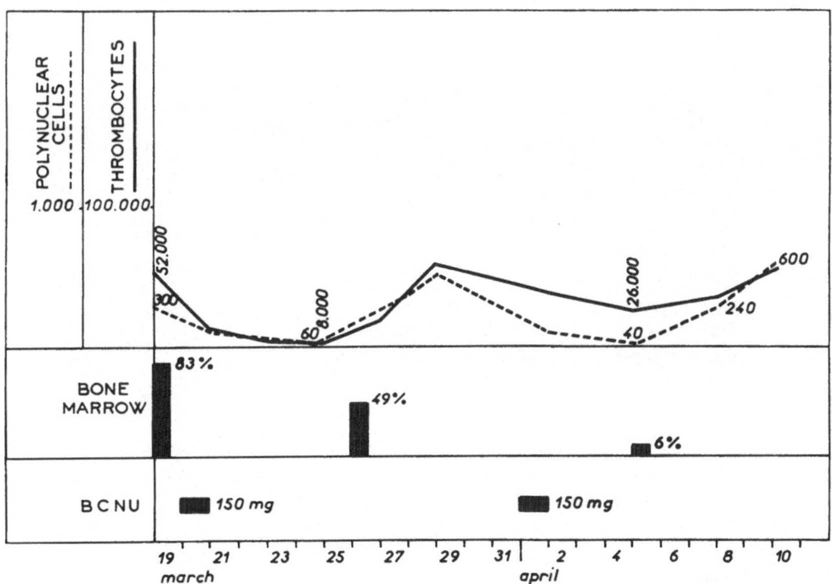

Fig. 5. Induction of a remission in acute lymphoblastic leukaemia with nitrosourea (BCNU)

mycin, adriamycin, nitroso-urea, asparaginase, ICRF 159 or 1,2-bis(3,5-dioxopiperazine-1-yl)propane).

Though there may be several active compounds in one pharmacological group, for example 6-mercaptopurine, thioguanine, and azathioprine in the antipurines, A-methopterine or methotrexate, aminopterine and dichloroamethopterine in the antifolates, in practice, only one drug from each group will be available, for, when

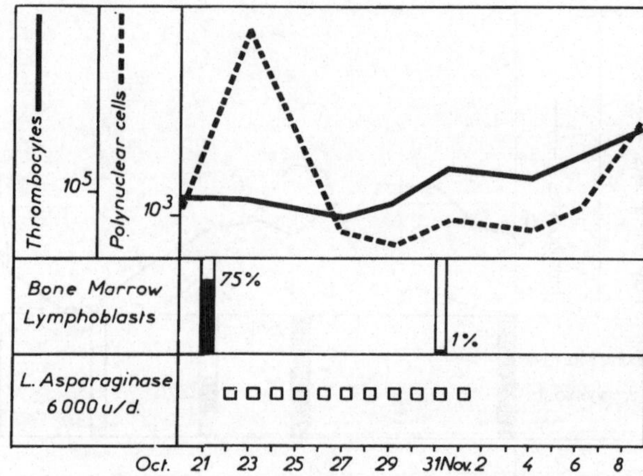

Fig. 6. Induction of a remission in acute lymphoblastic leukaemia with L-asparaginase

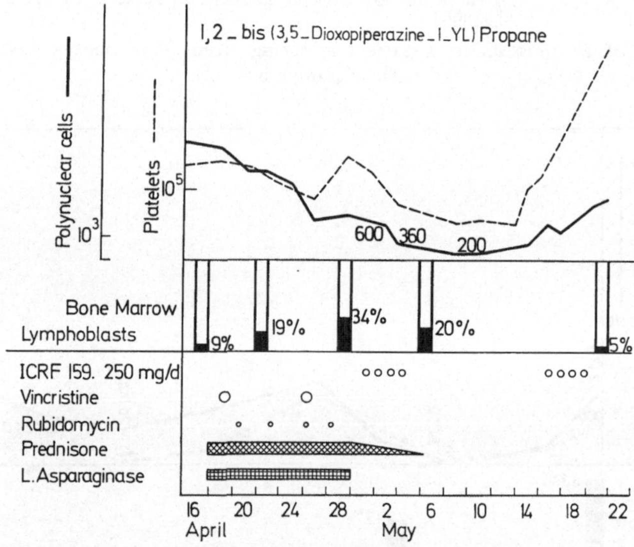

Fig. 7. Induction of a remission in acute lymphoblastic leukaemia with 1,2-bis(3,5-dioxopiperazine-1-yl)propane (ICRF 159) after the failure of therapy with leurocristine, rubidomycin, prednisone and L-asparaginase

a patient is resistant to one drug in a pharmacological group, he is resistant to all other products in this group.

On the other hand, when a patient is resistant to a given dose, he can be sensitive to a higher dose, this is illustrated in Fig. 8; the injection of methotrexate, 450 mg/m^2 for 48 hours once a week failed to check the proliferation of lymphoblastic leukaemia, but a remission was obtained when the dose was increased to 900 mg/m^2.

Table 1 has listed the drugs that are at present available for the treatment of acute lymphoblastic leukaemia, and their efficiency is estimated from their ability to induce remissions.

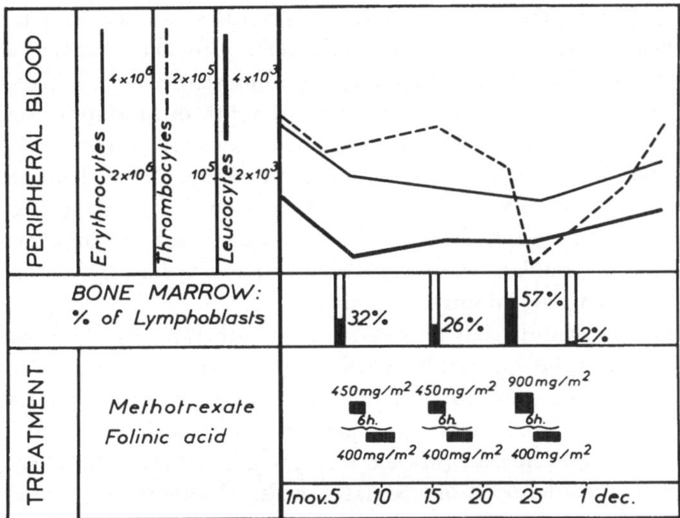

Fig. 8. Acute lymphoblastic leukaemia: failure of the combination of methotrexate in a dose (75 mg/m²/every 8 hours, for 48 hours) and folinic acid—rapid induction of remission with twice the dose of MTX

Methotrexate (5 mg/every second day) (WHITESIDE et al., 1958) and cytosine arabinoside (20 mg/every second day) can be injected into the cerebro-spinal fluid, and both these drugs effectively inhibit lymphoblastic proliferation in the meninges, which is a frequent complication of acute leukaemia.

The value of the drugs is not only judged by their ability to induce remissions. Certain of them, when appropriately administered, can prolong these remissions. Methotrexate (Ac. L. G. B., 1965), 6-mercaptopurine (FREIREICH et al., 1963) and cyclophosphamide (Ac. L. G. B., 1965), are generally considered to be the best chemotherapeutic agents for "maintenance" therapy. Their actions have been studied by comparative clinical trials.

2. *Radiotherapy* is used very much less than chemotherapy in the treatment of acute lymphoblastic leukaemia. We will see later that it can be usefully employed in certain clinical situations. Lymphoblastic leukaemias are very sensitive to radiotherapy, whether given in the form of local irradiation on mass causing symptoms, particularly in the mediastinum (D'ANGIO et al., 1959), or to cells localised in the nodes, testicle or meninges; the leukaemia has also been found to be sensitive when total body irradiation has been attempted, either in a sublethal dose (ANDREWS et al., 1961), or in a lethal dose followed by an isogeneic bone marrow transfusion from monozygotic twins (ATKINSON et al., 1959; THOMAS et al., 1959; MATHÉ et al., 1965), or followed by autologous marrow transfusion, taken during a remission (MCGOVERN et al., 1959). The tumour masses in lymphoblastic leukaemia generally disappear rapidly following local irradiation; remissions have been obtained following total body irradiation. It is true that total body irradiation greatly endangers the life of the patient, but it can be asked whether this risk is no more than that from certain forms of chemotherapy given at particular moments in the evolution of leukaemia.

3. *Surgery,* on the other hand, is only exceptionally indicated for the treatment of acute leukaemia. We have carried out splenectomy in some patients with splenomegaly, at certain stages in the disease, for reasons that we shall discuss later on. Enlargement of one testicle can be an indication for orchidectomy under certain conditions, especially if the abdominal lymphangiograms are normal.

4. *Immunotherapy* is the most recently introduced method for leukaemia therapy, and it looks as if it is capable of being greatly developed during the next few years. According to whether antibodies, immunocompetent cells (lymphocytes), or an attempt is made to stimulate the body's own immune defences, immunotherapy is called respectively, passive, adoptive or active.

a) Up until now, valid trials of *passive* immunotherapy have not been made in man. For such trials to be acceptable, it would be necessary to separate the cytotoxic antibodies, which would need to be given alone, from facilitation antibodies ("enhancement"). We have demonstrated in patients with choriocarcinoma, the reality of facilitation antibodies in man (MATHÉ et al., 1964; AMIEL et al., 1967), and these could enhance the proliferation of neoplastic cells. The results of studies at present being caried out by MOTTA (1969) allows us to hope that passive immunotherapy will eventually be able to be used as a method of destroying tumour cells.

b) *Adoptive* immunotherapy is based on the anti-tumour effect of the graft-versus-host reaction. We have demonstrated this anti-tumour effect by experiments on mice carrying the L 1210 grafted leukaemia (MATHÉ et al., 1959, 1962, 1968), CHARLOTTE FRIEND viral leukaemia (MATHÉ et al., 1962, 1964) and the spontaneous AkR leukaemia (MATHÉ et al., 1958, 1960). This method has the inconvenience of being complicated by the general effects of this graft-versus-host reaction, which show themselves in the form of the "secondary disease".

Good results with only slight risks can be obtained in certain model systems in experimental animals, where the lymphocyte donors can be specifically immunised against the tumour antigens (MATHÉ et al., 1969), but, at the present time, this system cannot be applied to man and attempts at an adoptive immunotherapy can only consist of a non-specific adoptive immunotherapy.

Remissions, generally of short duration, have been obtained in man by the *transfusion of allogeneic lymphocytes* (SCHWARZENBERG et al., 1965, 1966); very long remissions were obtained after *allogeneic bone marrow grafts* (due to the lymphocytes transferred by the graft proliferating in the host) (MATHÉ et al., 1959, 1960, 1963, 1965, 1968, 1968).

c) *Active* immunotherapy consists of the stimulation of the immune defences of the body against the tumour cells; it can be *non-specific,* consisting of the administration of immunological adjuvants, or *specific,* consisting of the administration of tumour antigens, by injecting tumour cells carrying these antigens that have been inactivated by irradiation *in vitro.*

We have shown in mice that immunotherapy can be effective even when it is given *after* the graft of L 1210 leukaemia (MATHÉ, 1968; MATHÉ et al., 1969). The important features of these experiments are as follows: a) tumour cells are generally immunotherapeutically more active than B. C. G., which is the best adjuvant we have so far discovered; b) the association of B. C. G. and tumour cells is more active than when each one of these is given alone; c) B. C. G. is more active if its administration is repeated several times, than when it is given as a single dose; leukaemic cells are just as active when they are given as a single dose as when they are repeated; d) the effective immunotherapy is so efficient that it can cause a complete regression of leukaemic cell proliferation and cure the animals; e) but, its effect, large or small, is only noticeable when 10^5 leukaemic cells or less have been grafted into the animal; it is totally ineffective on larger grafts.

We have confirmed this immunotherapeutic effect on two other tumours—the Rauscher transplantable leukaemia and the E ♀ K1 transplantable leukaemia (MATHÉ and POUILLART, 1970).

The use of active immunotherapy in man would only be justified if the human leukaemic cells carried new antigens, as had been detected in all animal cancers that have been studied. Research that we have been making with DORÉ and his collaborators (1967), using cytotoxicity, immunofluorescence, complement fixation, immune adherence and lymphocyte transformation tests, have demonstrated, in the serum of more than one-third of leukaemic patients, the presence of antibody active against their own leukaemic cells, and against cells of other patients.

Certain authors have suggested, as the result of studies of the spontaneous leukaemia in AkR mice, that patients suffering from acute leukaemia ought to be immunologically tolerant of their own tumour cells. We have collected, with DORÉ and his colleagues (1970), certain experimental findings which make us doubt the reality of the tolerance in spontaneous leukaemia of AkR mice; there has been no such demonstration of tolerance in human leukaemia, and ORBACH (1968) has shown that chemotherapy, using 6-mercaptopurine or methotrexate or cyclophosphamide is capable of breaking immune tolerance.

We shall discuss later, the results obtained in our first trials of the treatment of human lymphoblastic leukaemia by active immunotherapy, carried out precisely as our experimental results have suggested it should be done, in patients probably carrying a very small number of leukaemic cells.

Until now, we have used as adjuvants B. C. G. placed on an area of scarified skin, and corynebacterium parvum, injected intra-muscularly. We are now carrying out our first trials with poly AU. At present, specific immunotherapy is being attempted using the intra-dermal or subcutaneous injection of allogeneic leukaemic lymphoblasts irradiated *in vitro*.

II. The Strategy of Treatment with a View to Eradication of Leukaemia

A. In Chemo-sensitive Patients

There are plenty of drugs available to-day that enable a remission to be obtained in acute lymphoblastic leukaemia. Treatment should first commence with chemotherapy, except for those patients who are resistant to all available drugs. The first objective for the patient suffering from acute lymphoblastic leukaemia is the induction of a remission. Drugs must be chosen that give the patient the best chance to enter into this phase; the second objective is to attempt to cure the disease by trying to eradicate the leukaemic cell population.

a) The Induction of the Remission

Table 1 shows that though there are a number of drugs available to-day, which are capable of inducing remissions, the most effective of them, when given alone, (prednisone and vincristine) hardly give more than 50 per cent remissions, and the others only give 10 to 30 per cent.

The use of combinations of these drugs was tried to attempt to obtain a remission in all patients. Table 2 shows the high frequency of remissions obtained by the main combinations of drugs which have been the subject of clinical trial.

Table 2. *Value of various associations to induce remissions in acute lymphoblastic leukaemia*

Associations	% of complete remissions	References
Prednisone	84%	SELAWRY et al., 1965
(100 mg/m²/day) + vincristine	68%	Pers. exp. (not published)
Prednisone (100 mg/m²/day) + 6-mercaptopurine	82%	FREI, KARON et al., 1965
Prednisone (100 mg/m²/day) + methotrexate	80%	KRIVIT et al., 1966
Methotrexate + 6-mercaptopurine	45%	FREI et al., 1961
Prednisone + vincristine + methotrexate + 6-mercaptopurine	94%	FREIREICH et al., 1964
Prednisone (100 mg/m²/day) + vincristine	85% All visible phase and all ages	MATHÉ, HAYAT et al., 1967
+ rubidomycin	100% Children in 1st visible phase	

b) Attempts at Eradication of the Leukaemic Cell Population by Immunotherapy Preceded by a Complementary Cytoreductive Chemotherapy

Obtaining a remission alone does not cure the patient, it is known that if, after obtaining a remission, the patient receives no complementary therapy he is condemned to have an inevitable relapse. This relapse is due to the persistence of leukaemic cells. In patients with apparently complete remissions, as indicated by conventional examination, that is a normal blood count and a normal bone marrow, we have detected, on more detailed and cytological and histological examination, the presence of leukaemic cells in 17.5 per cent of these patients (MATHÉ et al., 1966). Abdominal lymphadenography systematically performed at this stage may

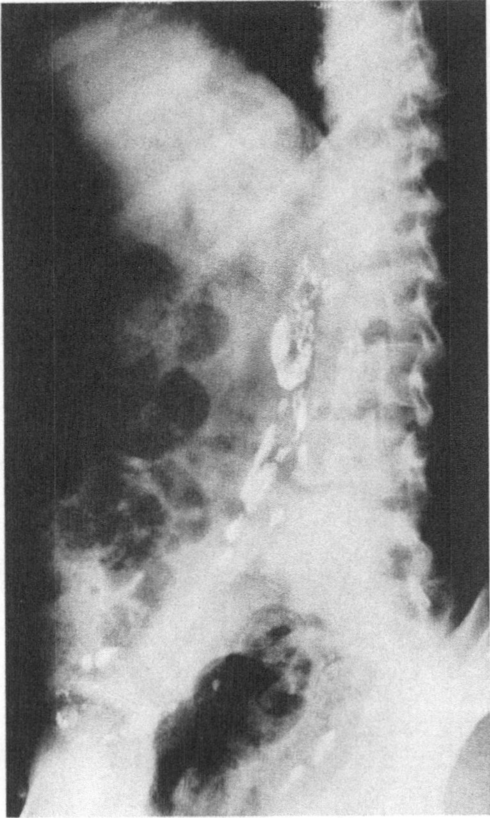

Fig. 9

Fig. 9 and 10. Lymphangiography showing the presence of peri-aortic adenopathies during an apparently complete remission in patient with acute lymphoblastic leukaemia

reveal persistance of adenopathy (Fig. 9 and 10). Taking the doubling time of A. L. L. to be four days, and if it is considered that the disease becomes visible when the child has a total of 10^{12} leukaemic cells in his body, then it can be calculated that following a remission induced by prednisone, 10^{8} cells will remain (FREI, 1964) and 10^{9} cells will remain after a remission induced by vincristine. In other words, the course of prednisone only destroys 99.99 per cent of the cells and vincristine only destroys 99.9 per cent.

Despite the hypothetical factor of these figures, they can act as a guide for the strategy of the overall treatment that is aimed to cure the patients: a) it is known that chemotherapy never destroys all the cells in the population, and can only destroy a given percentage: this phenomenon obeys the rules of first order kinetics; the drugs could not cure the patient unless his immune defences were able to destroy the remaining cells. We known that normal immune defences can only eradicate an extremely small number of tumour cells (in the order of 20 in the mouse), and we

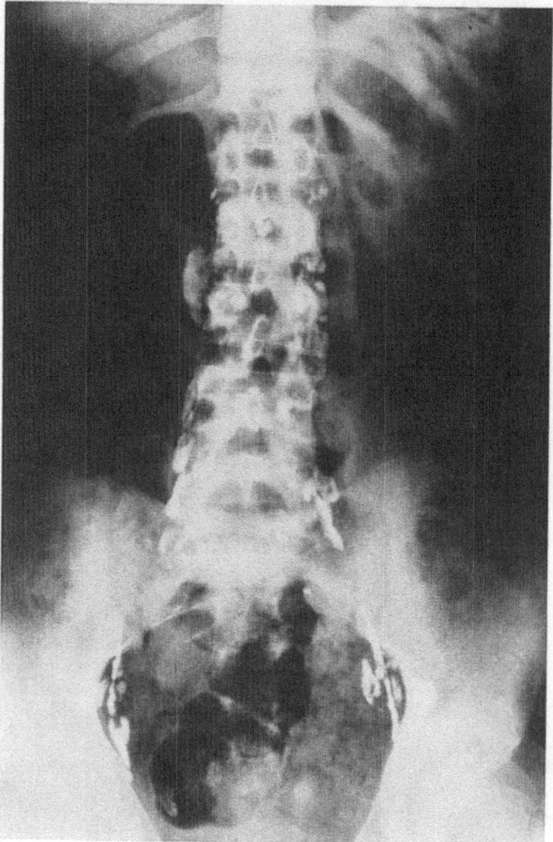

Fig. 10

know that the majority of drugs used in cancer chemotherapy, especially prednisone and 6-mercaptopurine, and in particular if they are given daily, are strongly immunosuppressive (see SCHNEIDER, 1968).

The hope of attaining a cure by using maintenance chemotherapy alone is, therefore, reduced. For as these drugs obey the rules of first order kinetics, it is difficult for them to reduce the number of leukaemic cells to a very low number so that the normal immune defences can eradicate them. If the immune defences were greatly weakened, as so often happens due to the immunosuppressive action of the drugs, then it would be impossible to eliminate completely the leukaemic cells.

In mice, where only about 20 cells can be eradicated by the normal immune defences, when these defences have been stimulated, even after a leukaemic graft, they can eliminate up to 10^5 cells (MATHÉ, 1968). These facts suggested the idea of applying successively to patients, a chemotherapy to induce remission which should, theoretically, lower the number of cells from 10^{12} to 10^8, a complementary cytoreductive chemotherapy to attempt to reduce the leukaemic population to a number that could be eradicated by immunotherapy and, finally, active immunotherapy.

c) Protocols of Treatment and their Results

Since 1964 we have carried out a number of different trials of therapy using various protocols of treatment for the investigation of the effect of chemotherapy and immunotherapy.

Protocols 1 and 2

Fig. 11 and 12 give the details of two schemes for the induction of remission and complementary cytoreductive chemotherapy.

The patients were also given intrathecal methotrexate (5 mg/week) and systematic radiation of the central nervous system to a total dose of 1,000 rads. At the end of either course of chemotherapy, patients were admitted into the immunotherapy trial; in this trial they were divided into four groups: a) a control group who received no further treatment after stopping chemotherapy; b) a second group who received every 7 days, B. C. G. applied as 2 ml of a suspension containing 75 mg of living bacterial per ml poured onto twenty scarifications, each 5 cm long (total length 1 metre); c) a third group received, every 7 days, a subcutaneous injection of 4×10^7 leukaemic lymphoblasts coming from a pool of cells taken from several patients (the cells for the first ten injections were treated with formol to inactivate any possible virus, the cells for the subsequent injections were irradiated *in vitro* with 4,000 rads; d) a fourth group, who received the B. C. G. and the leukaemic cells. The patients were distributed among these four groups at random.

The results demonstrated the effectiveness of active immunotherapy in man under the conditions of this trial: at the 130th day, out of the 20 patients given immunotherapy, 11 patients were still in remission, whilst all the control patients had relapsed. Furthermore, these results make us wonder if the therapeutic strategy based on the succession of a chemotherapeutic induction of remission, chemotherapeutic cytoreduction and active immunotherapy has been capable of eradicating the whole population of leukaemic cells in certain patients. At the present time, 4 other patients have had late relapses; 7 are still in perfect remission, 4 of them for more than one year after stopping chemotherapy; 4 for more than 2 years and 2 of them for more than 3 years (nearly 4 years in one patient) (Fig. 13) (MATHÉ et al., 1968, 1969).

There is no statistically significant difference between the group receiving B. C. G. alone, (5 relapses out of 8, one after stopping treatment), the group receiving leukaemic cells alone (3 relapses out of 5) and the group receiving B. C. G. and leukaemic cells (5 relapses out of 7).

It is of interest that the majority of patients given immunotherapy and who subsequently relapsed, did so early. This correlates with the results found in mice and suggests that in these patients, the number of cells which persisted after the arrest of chemotherapy was greater than the number that could be influenced by immunotherapy. Some of the late relapses that we have observed in man correspond to certain late relapses that we have also seen in mice; it is possible that sometimes the action of immunotherapy is limited to keeping the leukaemic cells in G_0 [3]. LHERITIER, SPEELMAN and BULENS (in preparation) have shown that, when the growth curve of a tumour treated with immunotherapy develops a plateau, the cells are not in G_0, and there is reason to believe that cell production and cell destruction are equal.

[3] Outside the cell cycle.

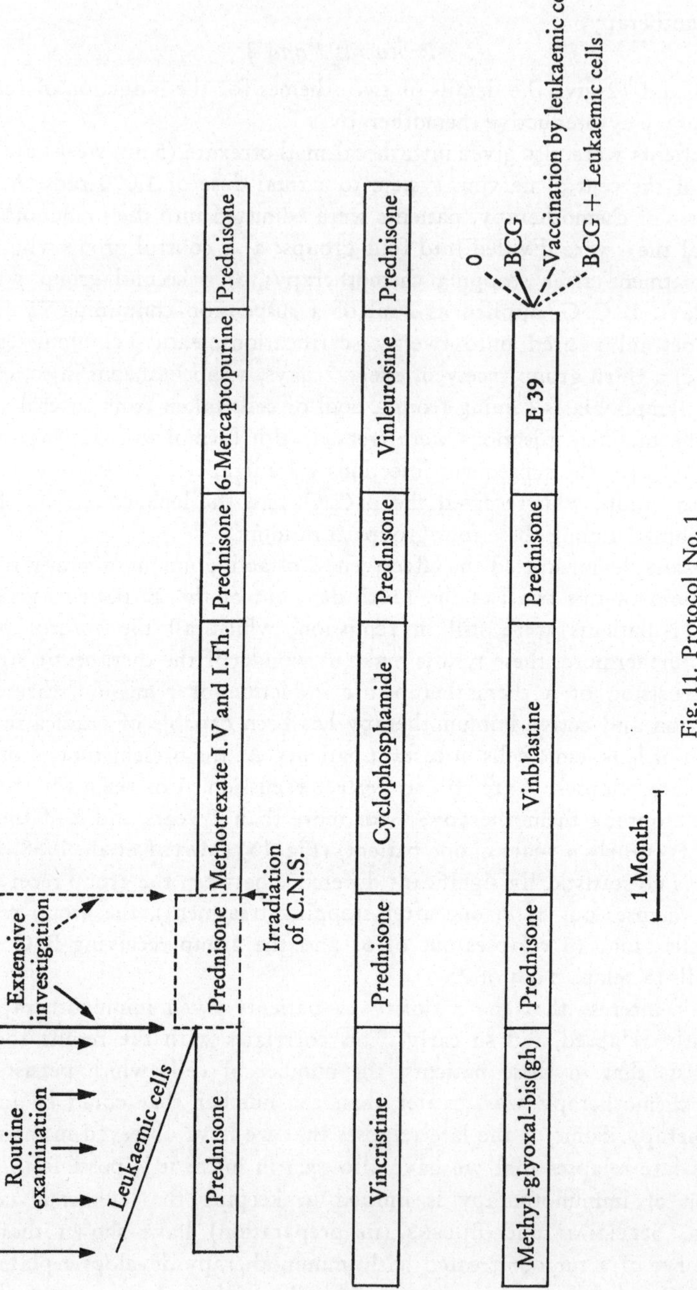

Fig. 11. Protocol No. 1

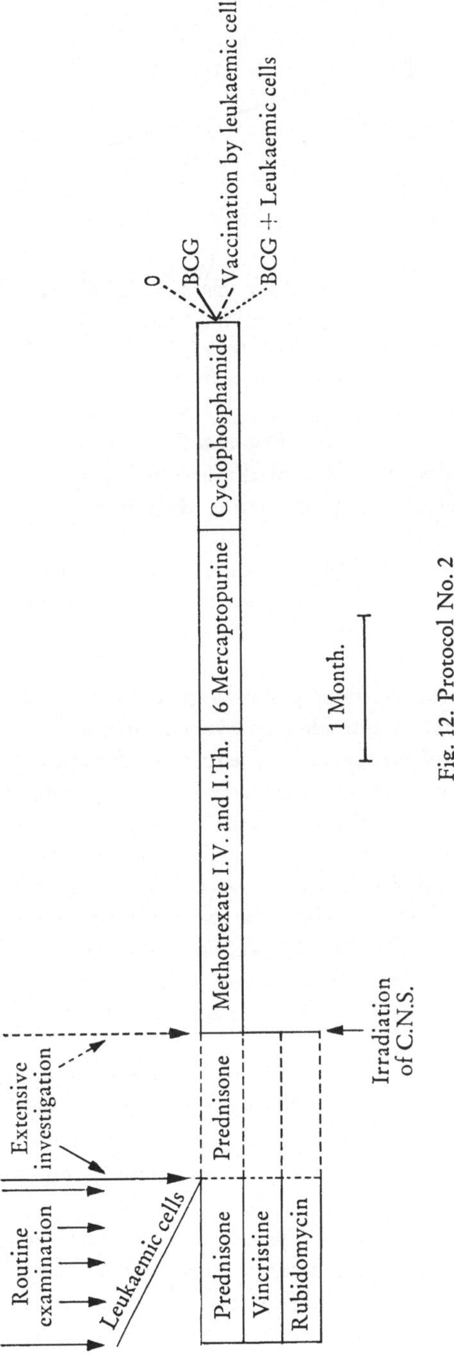

Fig. 12. Protocol No. 2

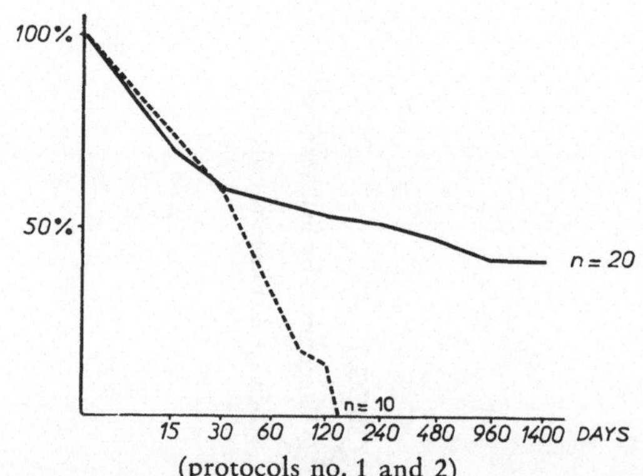

(protocols no. 1 and 2)

——— Patients submitted to immunotherapy; ---- patients without immunotherapy

Fig. 13. Actuarial curves of the duration of complete remissions after stopping chemotherapy

Protocol 5 [4]

Following the results of the use of the first two protocols, an attempt was made to make the complementary cytoreductive chemotherapy and the immunotherapy more effective.

A protocol was established in which the combination of drugs shown in Fig. 14 were given to the patients and then, following chemotherapy, they were divided into 3 groups at random. The first group received only active immunotherapy, being the injection of B. C. G., Corynebacterium parvum and irradiated leukaemic cells (our experiments in mice had previously shown that 1) the addition of two adjuvants, though it did not produce a notable improvement in the effect obtained with the best of either of them, it did not reduce the effect; 2) the addition of irradiated cells to the adjuvant gave a better result than when each was used alone). The patients in the second group were given the same immunotherapy and also received amantadine (100 mg/day in children, 200 mg/day in adults), an agent that is known to affect the replication of certain RNA viruses (OKER BLUM, personal communication); the patients in the third group were given the same immunotherapy and also received an injection of vincristine each month (we have not noticed any marked immunosuppressive effect as when this drug is given intermittently). Intrathecal injections of methotrexate were used in this protocol, but radiotherapy of the central nervous system was omitted.

The definite *results* of this trial are still not available, but it is already apparent that the complementary cytoreductive chemotherapy is unable to reduce in all the patients, the number of tumour cells to a number of cells that can be effectively eradicated by any supplementary treatment and already some meningeal relapses have occured.

It can be seen, in the legend of Fig. 15, that the duration of the complete remission, after the arrest of complementary cytoreductive chemotherapy, was longer in those patients who were given this protocol at the outset of their illness, compared to those who received it either in the course of a relapse or after a previous course of conventional chemotherapy.

[4] The third and fourth protocols were abandoned before they included a significant number of patients.

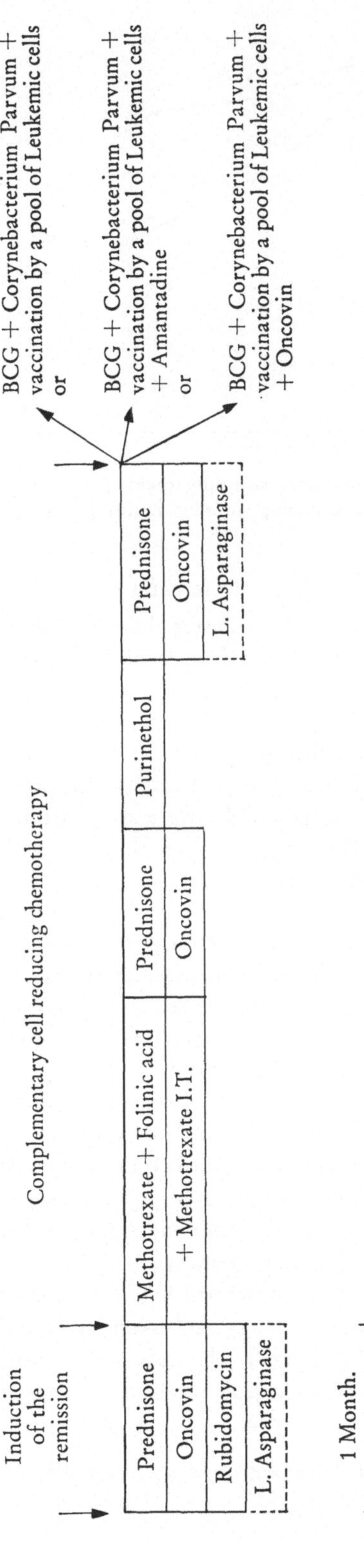

Fig. 14. Protocol No. 5

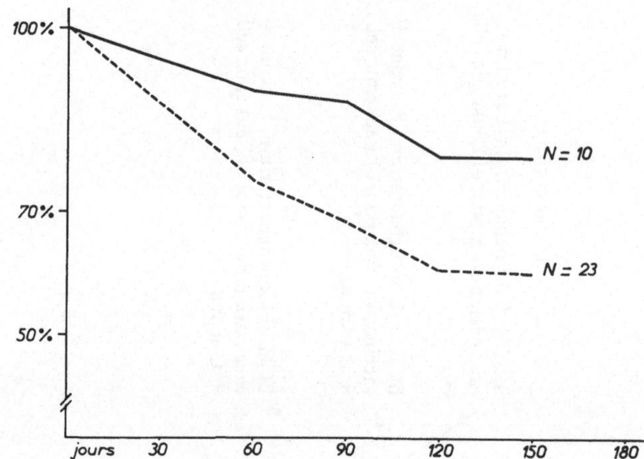

Fig. 15. Duration of remissions after stopping chemotherapy in patients treated according to protocol 5, during the first visible phase or a relapse

Protocol 6 [5]

One of the major theoretical criticisms that can be made of Protocol 5, as well as its predecessors, is that only one drug is given during the complementary cytoreductive chemotherapy phases. Since it is known that methotrexate and 6-mercaptopurine can only induce remissions in 50 per cent of the patients, it is to be feared there is a 1 in 2 chance that the number of tumour cells will increase during each of these phases. We have now set up a protocol which takes count of this criticism, in which at least two drugs are given during each phase of the complementary cytoreductive chemotherapy. The drugs used in this protocol are shown in Fig. 16. It will be noted that the chemotherapy to induce a remission only uses prednisone and vincristine. We have seen, in patients whose remission was induced by the combination of prednisone, vincristine and daunomycin, severe bone marrow aplasia at the time of commencing complementary chemotherapy. It is possible that daunomycin irreversibly affects the myeloid stem cells reducing their total number. Adriamycin is only given during the period of induction, to patients whose leukaemia is resistant to vincristine and prednisone (about 15 per cent).

The sequence in which the various drugs are given takes into account their immunosuppressive effects. The very immunosuppressive drugs are given initially and complementary chemotherapy is ended, using the combination of L-asparaginase and methotrexate, administered intermittently, which we have observed to have little or no immunosuppressive action. The immune reactions thereby have time to reappear before the commencement of immunotherapy.

We have also added to the intrathecal (i.t) injections of methotrexate, i.t. injections of cytosine-arabinoside (20 mg) and systematic radiotherapy of the central nervous system (1,000 rads). Finally, the patient is given local radiotherapy of all nodes or organs which were enlarged, and splenectomy if the spleen was enlarged during the visible phase of the disease.

[5] This protocol is called "Concord" and was established as a joint project with our collegues in England.

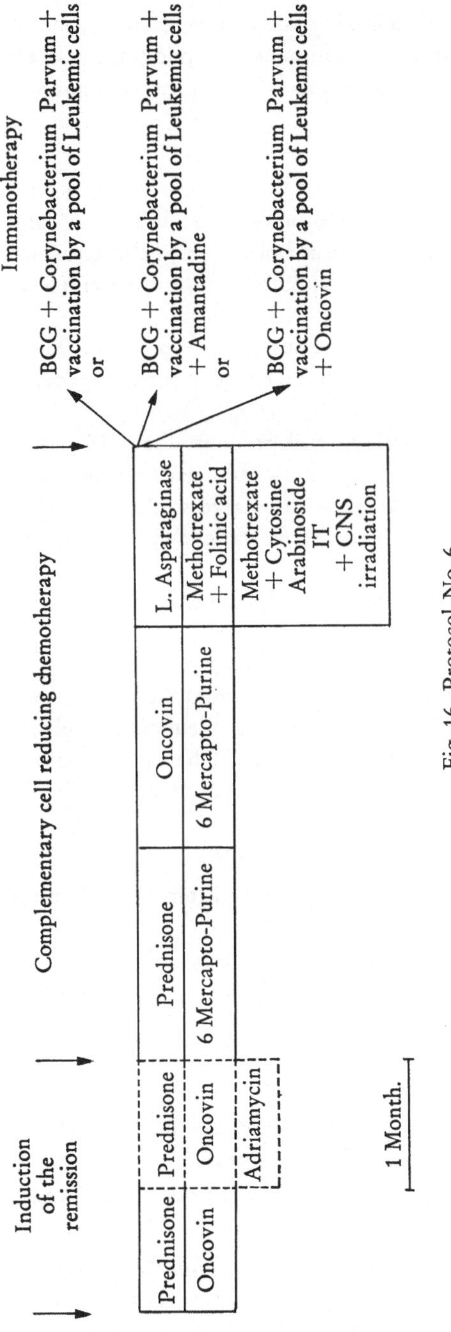

Fig. 16. Protocol No. 6

An extensive investigation is made at the end of the course of chemotherapy to induce a remission. This especially includes the counting, after leucoconcentration, of the blast cells in the peripheral blood (more than 40 per 10,000 nucleated cells is considered to be abnormal); abdominal lymphography is also carried out in these patients (Fig. 9 and 10). The details of this protocol that we are using at present is as follows:

Induction of Remission

An attempt to induce a remission is made using the combination of prednisone and vincristine (the patient can be at home during this treatment):

Prednisone: 40 mg/m²/day by mouth; it should be given in divided doses throughout the night and day.

Vincristine, 1.5 mg/m² intravenously, once a week. This treatment should continue for at least a month and about 85 per cent of apparently complete remissions will be obtained.

Should this treatment fail, as will occur in about 15 per cent of the patients, it is important to realise this as early as possible, as indicated by the failure of blast cells to diminish in the peripheral blood or marrow, then the combination of prednisone, vincristine and adriamycin is used (the patient must be admitted to hospital for this treatment):

Adriamycin: 10 mg/m²/day for 4 days intravenously; the first day should be the same day as the injection of vincristine.

Once an apparently complete remission has been obtained, the following investigations should be undertaken: blood count, bone marrow examination and leucoconcentration to estimate the number of leukaemic cells, electro-encephalogram, gammaencephalogram, lymphangiography (the lymphangiography can be deferred for several days or weeks if there is thrombocytopenia or neutropenia).

Complementary Cytoreductive Chemotherapy

This ought to be initiated immediately after the induction of a remission. There are three phases to this therapy:

a) *The first phase:* the patient being at home.

Prednisone: 40 mg/m²/day, by mouth, in divided equal doses throughout the day and night.

6-mercaptopurine, 70 mg/m²/day, by mouth, in divided doses during the day.

Duration, one and a half months.

b) *The second phase:* the patient should be admitted to hospital.

Vincristine: 0.5 mg/m²/week, intravenously.

6-mercaptopurine: 70 mg/m²/day, divided dose throughout the day.

Duration, one and a half months.

c) *The third phase:* the patient should be admitted to hospital.

L-asparaginase: 35,000 units/m²/day, intravenously, in two daily injections. If intravenous injections are impossible, they can be replaced by intramuscular injections.

Methotrexate: this can be given in one of two ways: 1) injection of 40 mg/m² intravenously or intramuscularly every 8 hours for 48 hours, making a total of 6 injections, then give folinic acid, 25 mg/m², i.v. or i.m., commencing 8 hours after the last injection of methotrexate, this is repeated 8-hourly for 4 days, making a total of 12 injections. 2) Injection of 15 mg/m^2, i.m. twice a week.

During this period, the following intrathecal treatment is given:

a) Intrathecal injections of methotrexate (5 mg) and cytosine arabinoside (20 mg): methotrexate is given first, following by the cytosine arabinoside 2 days later.

If these drugs are well tolerated, they can be injected simultaneously in the same doses as above: the patient should be given three injections per week for 6 weeks.

b) Radiotherapy of the meninges: at the end of the intrathecal chemotherapy, the patient is irradiated with a dose of 1,500 rads, to the whole of the meninges down to the level of the second sacral vertebrae.

At the end of the complementary cytoreductive chemotherapy, the extensive investigation of the patient should be repeated, with the exception that it will only be necessary to take pictures of the previously opacified lymph nodes.

Possible complementary treatment: if the patient had splenomegaly during the visible phase of the disease, the spleen should be removed. If the patient has any evidence of lymphadenopathy, as shown clinically or on lymphangiography, the nodes should be treated with a local radiation of 3,000 rads.

Supplementary Immunotherapy, with or without Anti-viral Therapy, with or without Chemotherapy

At this stage, the patients are divided into three groups, at random.

The first group: the patient receives every four days for a month and then once a week, the following combination:

BCG: 20 scratches are made on the skin, each 5 cm long, arranged in a square; into this is poured 2 ml of a suspension containing 75 mg of living bacteria (dry weight) per ml.

Corynebacterium parvum (reticulostimuline): a suspension of formolised Corynebacterium parvum is injected once a week: 750 µg in children and 1,250 µg in adults.

Vaccination with leukaemic lymphoblasts: the patient is given weekly, for three weeks, 4×10^7 leukaemic lymphoblasts treated with formol, then every 15 days for six weeks, followed by once a month, 4×10^7 lymphoblasts irradiated *in vitro* with a dose of 4,000 rads.

The second group: the patients in the second group received the same treatment as those in the first group and, in addition, they were given 100 mg (children) or 200 mg (adults) of amantadine per day.

The third group: the same treatment as the first group, but in one week out of four, the immunotherapy is replaced by an intravenous injection of vincristine, 1.5 mg/m^2.

B. Patients who are Chemo-Resistant

When the patients present a resistance to one of the drugs, as indicated by a relapse during its administration, this drug is eliminated from the protocol and a special protocol is set up. Two of the drugs used in combination can be replaced by associations of drugs which have not been utilised in the protocol for chemo-sensitive patients. The following combinations can be used: nitrosourea (BCNU) (100 mg/m^2 per day, once a week intravenously) and cytosine arabinoside (50 mg/m^2 every 3 hours for 24 hours, intravenously, repeated every fourth day); cyclophosphamide (600 mg/m^2

per week, intramuscularly or i.v.) and cytosine arabinoside in the same dose as given above; or methyl-glyoxal-bis(guanylhydrazone) (100 mg/m^2, 3 times a week intravenously) and nitrosourea (as above).

Should the patient be resistant to all forms of chemotherapy, a remission can be obtained by *adoptive immunotherapy*, using *lymphocyte transfusions* (Schwarzenberg et al., 1965, 1966). Unfortunately, these remissions are of short duration.

Remission can still be obtained using *total body irradiation*, either in a sublethal dose or a lethal dose. Irradiation should be followed, in the latter case, by an *autologous transfusion of bone marrow* [taken previously during a state of remission, and stored at $-70°$ C or at $-190°$ C (McGovern et al., 1959)], or *isogeneic marrow*, if the patient has a homozygous twin (Thomas et al., 1959; Mathé et al., 1965).

Total body irradiation at a lethal dose, followed by a *marrow allograft* which combines the effects of irradiation and adoptive immunotherapy, replacing the marrow of the patient with a healthy marrow is still only at an experimental stage and carries the risk of secondary disease which is the consequence of the reaction of the graft against the host (Mathé et al., 1968).

The possibility of preparing the recipients with cyclophosphamide instead of irradiation (Santos, 1970) may make this method of treatment more applicable.

We have recently successfully grafted allogeneic bone marrow after simply conditioning the patient with antilymphocyte serum (Mathé et al., 1968). This new technique will possibly allow the indications for marrow transplantations to be increased.

III. Symptomatic Treatment

During the visible phases of the illness, the patient is submitted to the risks of myeloid insufficiency, leading to anaemia, neutropenia and infection, thrombocytopenia and haemorrhage.

Red cell transfusions are indicated if the anaemia is very marked: they are useless if the anaemia is not profound and they are even dangerous, for they can immunise the patient and may jeopardise the value of later white cell or bone marrow transfusions. *Platelet transfusions* are very important in the case of severe thrombocytopenia (Schwarzenberg et al., 1966), and *transfusions of granulocytes* are of value in neutropenia complicated by septicaemia (Schwarzenberg et al., 1966, 1966). Antibiotics should be used as indicated by bacteriological testing, but they are generally ineffective in the case of septicaemia or patients who have profound neutropenia (Schneider, 1967). Transfusions of granulocytes are frequently effective in this condition (Fig. 17).

Granulocyte transfusions allow chemotherapy, even a drug or a combination that causes myeloid aplasia, to be given to a patient who is already aplasic. Normally, this practice would be avoided due to the risk of making the aplasia worse and the leukaemia would proliferate unchecked. With granulocyte transfusions, the chemotherapy can be given without risk and possibly induces a remission, as is shown in Table 3 and Fig. 18 (Schwarzenberg et al., 1969).

Nursing patients in pathogen free rooms, of the type that we have used at the Institut de Cancérologie et d'Immunogénétique (Hopital Paul-Brousse) for the past five years, gives the severely neutropenic patient a remarkable protection from infec-

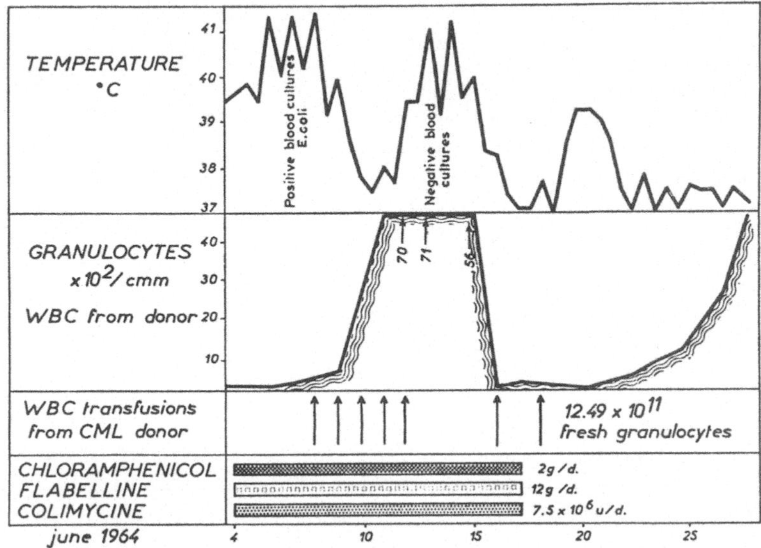

Fig. 17. Acute lymphoblastic leukaemia: Septicaemia resistant to antibiotics, that were active in vitro. The septicaemia was only able to be cured after transfusions of granulocytes

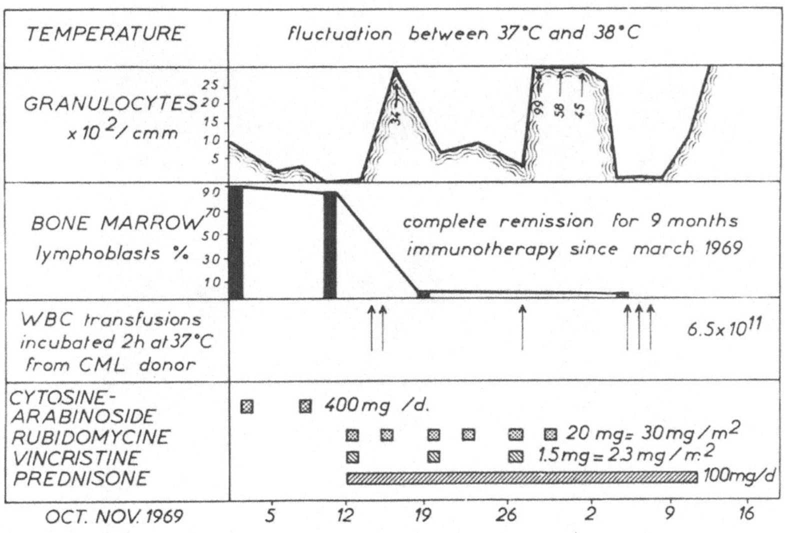

Fig. 18. Acute lymphoblastic leukaemia: a complete remission was obtained in one week with the combination of prednisone, rubidomycin and vincristine under the cover of leucocyte transfusions. Cytosine arabinoside had previously failed

tion (MATHÉ and FORESTIER, 1965; SCHNEIDER et al., 1969) (Fig. 19). This treatment may be indicated not only during the visible phase of the disease but also during the complementary cytoreductive chemotherapy phase, should it be followed by aplasia, a rare but possible event.

Table 3. *Chemotherapy of acute leukaemia patients with a neutrophil count < 800/cmm owing to protection by white blood cell transfusions*

		Complete remission	Incomplete remission	Total failure
Acute lymphoblastic leukaemia	Prednisone (100 mg/m²/day) Vincristine (1.5 mg/m²/day) Rubidomycin (20 mg/m²/twice a week)	6		2
	Cytosine arabinoside (50 mg/m²/3h×8 every 4th day)	1		1
	Methotrexate (75 mg/m²/8h×6) Folinic acid (25 mg/m²/6h×16)	2		
Acute myeloblastic leukaemia	Prednisone + vincristine + rubidomycin + methyl-GAG (200 mg/m²/every 2nd day)	1		
	Rubidomycin (80 mg/m²/4 days)		1	
Acute monoblastic leukaemia	Prednisone + vincristine + rubidomycin			1
	Cytosine arabinoside			1

No infectious complications in any patients.

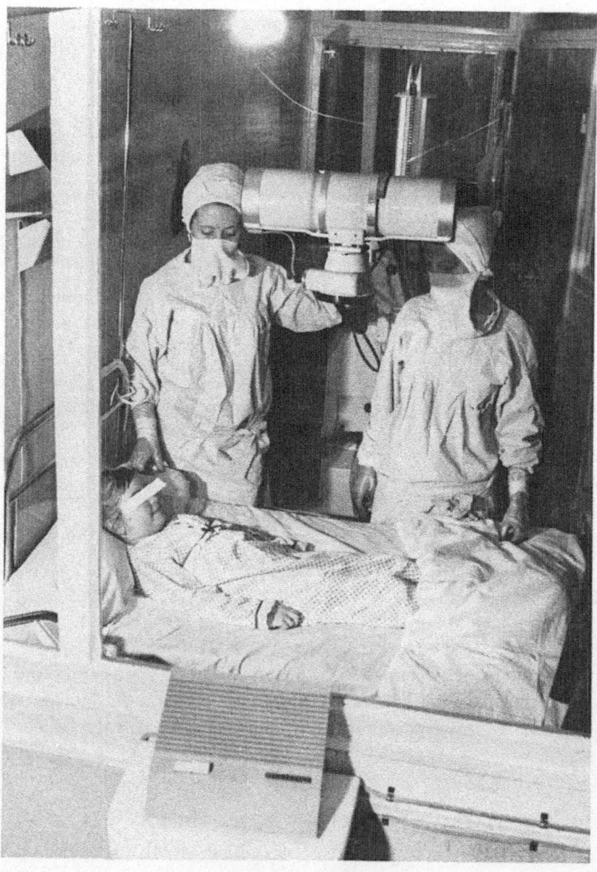

Fig. 19. One of the five pathogen-free rooms available at the "Institut de Cancérologie et d'Immunogénétique" (Villejuif)

Conclusions and Perspectives

The importance of specialised intensive care is high-lighted (SCHWARZENBERG et al., 1966, 1966) for, at one time or another during the illness, the state of the patient may necessitate a period of isolation in a pathogen-free room, leucocyte or platelet transfusion, and even a bone marrow graft.

The urgency of the requirement for treatment is stressed. The doubling time of the leukaemic cell is four days—that means if there is 4 days' delay in establishing a diagnosis or starting treatment, the tumour will have doubled in size. We have seen the importance of these quantitative factors in the results of therapy.

Scientifically designed treatments for the eradication of leukaemia have the best chance of being effective when they are started very early in the disease. We have seen, in patients treated according to our protocol 5, that less favourable results are obtained in patients who have been treated previously by conventional therapy than in those given the treatment at the onset of the first visible phase (Fig. 15).

Only a few cancers are treated from their outset by a scientifically based chemotherapeutic regime. In disseminated cancer, it is only rarely that the patient's chances will be impaired by a non-specialist physician instituting treatment of his own choice. However, just as in choriocarcinoma, where the chances of a cure are high if the patient is given effective therapy, it is likely that patients with A. L. L. will only have a chance of a long survival, or even a cure, when a scientifically proven treatment is instituted, and their chance will be higher if the treatment is started very early.

In an article entitled "Who should treat patients suffering from acute leukaemia?", JAMES HOLLAND (1969) gave an urgent message to physicians that, in the opinion of all specialists, procrastination in initiating the "best treatment" can profoundly influence the prognosis.

Summary

A.L.L. because of the easy quantification of the tumour volume, is a good model for the study of a scientific strategy for cancer treatment.

The methods available are the same as for any cancer: surgery, radiotherapy, chemotherapy and immunotherapy. The limits of their respective actions are clear: surgery is only useful for eradicating a local tumoral mass, whether detectable or not; radiotherapy for attempting to eradicate such a mass, success being proportional to radiosensitivity; chemotherapy is able to kill tumour cells in most parts of the body, but it obeys the first law of kinetics, e. g. it only destroys a certain percentage of the tumour cell population, never 100%; adoptive immunotherapy is not yet routinely operational; active immunotherapy is able to destroy a whole tumour population, but only if the number of its population is very small, of the order of 10^5: its action and its condition of action have been demonstrated by the authors of this paper, both with animal experiments and with a clinical trial in A.L.L.

Hence a therapeutic strategy is proposed combining (1) chemotherapy to reduce the number of the tumour cells as much as possible, (2) surgery and radiotherapy to eradicate any tumour mass persisting in certain areas poorly accessible to chemotherapy and immunotherapy, (3) active immunotherapy to eradicate the last few cells, provided the other treatments have reduced the original population to a sufficiently small number.

The results of a first trial conducted by the authors and protocols for the trials in progress are described.

References

Acute Leukemia Group B: New treatment schedule with improved survival in childhood leukemia. J. Amer. med. Ass. **194**, 75 (1965).

AMIEL, J. L., MERY, A. M., MATHÉ, G.: Les réponses immunitaires chez les patients atteintes de choriocarcinome placentaire. Corrélation entre ces réponses et l'évolution de la maladie, p. 197. In: C. R. Col. on «immunosuppression hématologique». Liège 1967.

ANDREWS, G. A., SITTERSON, B. W., KRETCHMAR, A. L., TANIDA, R.: Studies of total body irradiation and attempted marrow transplantation in acute leukemia. Acta haemat. (Basel) **26**, 129 (1961).

ANGIO, G. L. D', FARBER, S., MADDOCK, C. L.: Potentiation of X-ray effects by actinomycin D. Radiology **73**, 175 (1959).

ATKINSON, J. B., MAHONEY, J. F., SCHWARTZ, I. R., HESCH, J. A.: Therapy of acute leukemia by whole body irradiation and bone marrow transplantation from an identical twin. Blood **14**, 228 (1959).

BERNARD, J., BOIRON, M., JACQUILLAT, C., WEIL, M.: Un nouvel agent actif dans le traitement des leucémies aigues: la cytosine arabinosine. Presse méd. **74**, 799 (1966).

— WEIL, M., LEVY, J. P., SELIGMAN, M., NAJEAN, Y.: Etude de la rémission complète des leucémies aigues. Nouv. Rev. franç. Hémat. **2**, 195 (1962).

BONADONNA, G., MONFARDINI, S., DE LENA, M., FOSSATI-BELLANI, F.: Clinical evaluation of adriamycin, a new antitumour antibiotic. Brit. med. J. **3**, 503 (1969).

BURCHENAL, J. H., KARNOFSKY, D. A., MURPHY, M. L., OETTGEN, H. F.: Effects of L-asparaginase on leukemias and other neoplasms. In: XIIth congress int. Soc. Hemat. New York 1968, p. 7.

— MURPHY, M. L., ELLISON, R. R., SYKES, M. P., TAN, C. T., LEONE, L. A., KARNOFSKY, D. A., CRAVER, L. F., DARGEON, H. W., RHOADS, C. P.: Clinical evaluation of a new antimetabolite, 6-mercaptopurine, in the treatment of leukemia and allied diseases. Blood **8**, 965 (1953).

DORÉ, J. F., AJURIA, E., MATHÉ, G.: Non-leukaemic Arr mice are not tolerant to cells of leukaemia induced by Gross virus. Europ. J. clin. biol. Res. **15**, 81 (1970).

— MOTTA, R., MARHOLEV, L., HRSAK, Y., COLAS DE LA NOUE, H., SÉMAN, G., DE VASSAL, F., MATHÉ, G.: Preliminary results of research for new antigens in human leukemic cells and antibody in the serum of leukemic patients. Lancet **1967 II**, 1396.

FARBER, S., DIAMOND, L. K., MERCER, R. D., SYLVESTER, R. J., JR., WOLF, J. A.: Temporary remissions in acute leukemia in children produced by folic acid antagonist, 4-aminopteroylglutamic acid (aminopterin). New Engl. J. Med. **238**, 787 (1948).

FERNBACH, D. J., SUTOW, W. W., THURMAN, W. G., VIETTI, T. J.: Clinical evaluation of cyclophosphamide. A new agent for the treatment of children with acute leukemia. J. Amer. med. Ass. **182**, 30 (1962).

FREI, E. III.: Potential for eliminating leukemic cells in childhood acute leukemia. Proc. Amer. Ass. Cancer Res. **5**, 20 (1964).

— FREIREICH, E. J., GEHAN, E. A., PINKEL, D., HOLLAND, J. F., SELAWRY, O., HAURANI, F., SPURR, C. L., HAYES, D. M., JAMES, G. W., ROTHBERG, H., SODEE, D. B., RUNDLES, R. W., SCHROEDER, L. R., HOOGSTRATEN, B., WOLMAN, I. J., TRAGGIS, D. G., COOPER, T., GENDEL, B. R., EBAUGH, F., TAYLOR, R.: Studies of sequential and combination antimetabolite therapy in acute leukemia: 6-mercaptopurine and methotrexate (from the acute leukemia group B). Blood **18**, 431 (1961).

— KARON, M., LEVIN, R., FREIREICH, E. J., TAYLOR, R. J., HANANIAN, J., SELAWRY, O., HOLLAND, J. F., HOOGSTRATEN, B., WOLMAN, I. J., ABIR, E., SAWITSKY, A., LEE, S., MILLS, S. D., BURGET, O., JR., SPURR, C. L., PATTERSON, R. B., EBAUGH, F. G., JAMES, G. W., MOON, J. H.: The effectiveness of combinations of antileukemic agents in inducing and maintaining remission in children with acute leukemia. Blood **26**, 642 (1965).

FREIREICH, E. J., GEHAN, E. A., FREI, E. III., SCHROEDER, L. R., WOLMAN, I. J., AMBARI, R., BURGER, O., ILLS, S. D., PINKEL, D., SELAWRY, O. S., MOON, J. H., GENDEL, B. R., SPURR, C., STORES, R., HOURANI, F., HOOGSTRATEN, B., LEE, S.: The effect of 6-mercaptopurine on the duration of steroid induced remission in acute leukemia: a model of evaluation of other potentially useful therapy. Blood **21**, 699 (1963).

FREIREICH, E. J., KARON, M., FREI, E. III.: Quadruple combination therapy (VAMP) for acute lymphocytic leukemia of childhood. Proc. Amer. Ass. Cancer Res. **5**, 20 (1964).

HELLMAN, K.: Further clinical experiences with ICRF 159. Plenary session of the O.E.R.T.C., Paris, Vol. 1. Springer 1969 (in press).

HENDERSON, E. A., BURKE, P. J.: Clinical experience with cytosine arabinoside. Proc. Amer. Ass. Cancer Res. **6**, 26 (1965).

HILL, J. M., ROBERTS, J., LOEB, E., KHAN, A., HAYTON, M., HILL, R. W.: L-asparaginase therapy for treatment of leukemias and other malignant neoplasms. J. Amer. med. Ass. **202**, 882 (1967).

HOLLAND, J. F.: Who should treat acute leukemia? J. Amer. med. Ass. **209**, 1511 (1969).

JACQUILLAT, C., NAJEAN, Y., WEIL, M., TANZER, J., BOIRON, M., BERNARD, J.: Traitement des leucémies aigues lymphoblastiques par la rubidomycine. Path. et Biol. **15**, 913 (1967).

KRIVIT, N., BRUBAKER, C., HARTMANN, J., MURPHY, M. L., PIERCE, M., THATCHER, G.: Induction of remission in acute leukemia of childhood by combination of prednisone and either 6-mercaptopurine or methotrexate. J. Pediat. **68**, 965 (1966).

LHERITIER, J., BULENS, C., SPEELMAN, P.: to be published.

MACGOVERN, J. J., JR., RUSSEL, P. J., ATKINS, L., WEBSTER, E. W.: Treatment of terminal leukemia by total body irradiation and intravenous infusion of stored autologous bone marrow obtained during remission. New Engl. J. Med. **260**, 675 (1959).

MATHÉ, G.: Immunothérapie active de la leucémie L 1210 appliquée après la greffe tumorale. Rev. franç. Étud. clin. biol. **13**, 881 (1968).

— AMIEL, J. L.: Réduction de la concentration plasmatique du virus de Charlotte Friend par immunothérapie adoptive (greffe de moelle osseuse allogénique). C. R. Acad. Sci. **259**, 4408 (1964).

— — BERNARD, J.: Traitement de souris AkR à l'âge de 6 mois par irradiation totale suivie de transfusion de cellules hématopoïétiques. Incidences respectives de la leucémie et du syndrome secondaire. Bull. Cancer **47**, 331 (1960).

— — FRIEND, CH.: Essai de traitement de la leucémie de Charlotte Friend par la greffe de cellules hématopoïétiques de donneurs isogéniques vaccinés contre le virus. Bull. Cancer **49**, 416 (1962).

— — HAYAT, M., SCHWARZENBERG, L., SCHNEIDER, M., CATTAN, A., SCHLUMBERGER, J. R., CEOARA, B.: Essai de traitement de leucémies aigues et de la maladie de Hodgkin par la rubidomycine seule ou en association. Sem. Hôp. Paris **43**, 2109 (1967).

— — — VASSAL, F. DE, SCHWARZENBERG, L., SCHNEIDER, M., JASMIN, C., ROSENFELD, C.: Preliminary data on acute leukemia with ICRF 159. Plenary session of the E.O.R.T.C., Paris, Vol. 1. Springer 1969 (in press).

— — NIEMETZ, J.: Greffe de moelle osseuse après irradiation totale chez des souris leucémiques suivie de l'administration d'un antimitotique pour réduire la fréquence d'un syndrome secondaire et ajouter à l'effet antileucémique. C. R. Acad. Sci. **254**, 3603 (1962).

— — SCHWARZENBERG, L.: L'aplasie myélo-lymphoïde de l'irradiation totale, Vol. A. Ed.: GAUTHIER-VILLARS. Paris 1965.

— — — Bone marrow transplantation. In: Human transplantation, Vol. 1. New York: Grune & Stratton 1968, p. 284.

— — — CATTAN, A., SCHNEIDER, M.: Haematopoietic chimera in man after allogeneic (homologous) bone marrow transplantation: control of the secondary syndrome, specific tolerance due to chimerism. Brit. med. J. **2**, 1633 (1963).

— — — — — DE VRIES, M. J., TUBIANA, M., LALANNE, C., BINET, J. L., PAPIERNIK, M., SÉMAN, G., MATSUKURA, M., MERY, A. M., SCHWARZMANN, V., FLAISLER, A.: Successful allgeneic bone marrow transplantation in man: chimerism induced specific tolerance and possible antileukemic effects. Blood **25**, 179 (1965).

— — — SCHNEIDER, M., CATTAN, A., SCHLUMBERGER, J. R., HAYAT, M., DE VASSAL, F.: Démonstration de l'efficacité de l'immunothérapie active dans la leucémie aigue lymphoblastique. Rev. franç. Étud. clin. biol. **13**, 454 (1968).

— — — — CATTAN, A., SCHLUMBERGER, J. R., HAYAT, M., DE VASSAL, F.: Active immunotherapy for acute lymphoblastic leukemia. Lancet **1**, 697 (1969).

Mathé, G., Amiel, J. L., Schwarzenberg, L., Schneider, M., Cattan, A., Schlumberger, J. R., Hayat, M., De Vassal, F., Jasmin, C., Rosenfeld, C.: Essai de traitement de la leucémie aigue lymphoblastique par la L-asparaginase. Presse méd. **77**, 461 (1969).

— — — — — — — — — — — Choay, J., Trolard, P.: Greffe de moelle osseuse allogénique chez l'homme prouvée par 6 marqueurs antigéniques après conditionnement du receveur et du donneur par le sérum antilymphocytaire. Rev. franç. Étud. clin. biol. **13** 1025 (1968).

— Bernard, J.: Essai de traitement par l'irradiation X suivie de greffe de cellules myéloïdes homologues de souris atteintes de leucémie spontanée très avancée. Bull. Cancer **45**, 289 (1958).

— — Essai de traitement de la leucémie greffée L 1210 par l'irradiation X suivie de transfusion de cellules hématopoïétiques normales (isologues ou homologues, myéloïdes ou lymphoïdes, adultes ou embryonnaires). Rev. franç. Étud. clin. biol. **4**, 442 (1959).

— — Schwarzenberg, L., Larrieu, M. J., Lalanne, C., Dutreix, A., Denoix, P., Surmont, J., Schwarzmann, V., Ceoara, B.: Essai de traitement de sujets atteints de leucémie aigue en rémission par irradiation totale suivie de transfusions de moelle osseuse homologue. Rev. franç. Étud. clin. biol. **4**, 675 (1959).

— — De Vries, M. J., Schwarzenberg, L., Larrieu, M. J., Lalanne, C., Dutreix, A., Amiel, J. L., Surmont, J.: Nouveaux essais de greffe de moelle osseuse homologue après irradiation totale chez des enfants atteints de leucémie aigue en rémission. Le problème du syndrome secondaire chez l'homme. Rev. Hémat. **15**, 115 (1960).

— Dausset, J., Hervet, E., Amiel, J. L., Colombani, J., Brule, G.: Immunological studies in patients with placental choriocarcinoma. J. nat. Cancer Inst. **33**, 103 (1964).

— Forestier, P.: Un outil moderne de la recherche médicale française, l'Institut de Cancérologie et d'Immunogénétique. Intrications de la recherche expérimentale et clinique. Conditionnement hyposeptique des animaux et des malades. Techn. hosp. **20**, 47 (1965).

— Hayat, M., Schwarzenberg, L., Amiel, J. L., Schneider, M., Cattan, A., Schlumberger, J. R., Jasmin, C.: The high rate and quality of remissions induced by the combination of prednisone, vincristine and rubidomycin in acute lymphoblastic leukemia. The value of pathogen free rooms. Lancet **2**, 380 (1967).

— Pouillart, P.: Active immunotherapy of L 1210 leukemia applied after the graft of tumor cells. Brit. J. Cancer **423**, 814 (1969).

— — Active immunotherapy of mouse RC 19 and E ♀ k, leukaemia applied after the I-V-transplantation of the tumour cells. Europ. Rev. clin. biol. Res. **15** (in press).

— — Schwarzenberg, L.: Transfusions of lymphocytes from non immunized or immunized donors in mice leukemia therapy. Colloque sur les transfusions de globules blancs. Paris: C.N.R.S. 1969 (in press).

— Schwarzenberg, L.: Immunothérapie adoptive locale de la leucémie L 1210 ascitique. Analyse des facteurs de son efficacité. J. Europ. Cancer **4**, 211 (1968).

— — Amiel, J. L., Schneider, M., Cattan, A., Schlumberger, J. R.: Traitement de la leucémie aigue lymphoblastique pendant une rémission par l'irradiation du système nerveux central et l'administration successive de cures de 8 composés chimiothérapiques. Sem. Hôp. Paris **42**, 2960 (1966).

— — Mery, A. M., Cattan, A., Schneider, M., Amiel, J. L., Schlumberger, J. R., Poisson, J., Wajcner, G.: An extensive histological survey of patients with acute leukemia in complete remission. Brit. med. J. **1**, 640 (1966).

— — De Vries, M. J., Amiel, J. L., Cattan, A., Schneider, M., Binet, J. L., Tubiana, M., Lalanne, C., Nordmann, R., Schwarzmann, V.: Les divers aspects du syndrome secondaire compliquant les transfusions de moelle osseuse ou de leucocytes allogéniques chez des sujets atteints d'hémopathies malignes. Europ. J. Cancer **1**, 75 (1965).

— Schweisguth, O., Brule, G., Brezin, C., Amiel, J. L., Schwarzenberg, L., Schneider, M., Cattan, A., Jasmin, C., Smadja, R.: Essai de traitement par la leurocristine de la leucémie aigue lymphoblastique et du lymphoblastosarcome. Presse méd. **71**, 529 (1963).

— — — Schneider, M., Amiel, J. L., Schwarzenberg, L., Cattan, A.: Essai de traitement par la cyclophosphamide de la leucémie aigue lymphoblastique et du lymphoblastosarcome. Presse méd. **71**, 402 (1963).

— Séman, G.: Aspects histologiques et cytologiques des leucémies et hématosarcomes, Vol. 1. Éd.: Maloine. Paris 1963.

Motta, R.: The passive immunotherapy of murine leukemias. I. The production of antisera against leukemic neoantigens. Europ. J. clin. biol. Res. **15**, 161 (1970).

Oker Blum: Personal Communication.

Orvach-Arbouys, S.: Rupture de tolérance immunitaire par certains cytostatiques utilisés en chimiothérapie anticancéreuse. Rev. franç. Étud. clin. biol. **13**, 1014 (1968).

Santos, G. W.: Preparation of a recipient for a transplant by cyclophosphamide. Commun. Symp. on Bone marrow grafting. Paris, June 1969.

Schneider, M.: Les infections bactériennes et fungiques au cours des leucémies aigues. Sem. Hôp. Paris **43**, 438 (1966).

— Effet des chimiothérapies sur une réaction d'hypersensibilité (BCG). Rev. franç. Étud. clin. biol. **13**, 877 (1968).

— Schwarzenberg, L., Amiel, J. L., Cattan, A., Schlumberger, J. R., Hayat, M., De Vassal, F., Jasmin, C., Rosenfeld, C., Mathé, G.: Pathogenfree isolation unit. Three years' experience. Brit. med. J. **1**, 836 (1969).

Schwarzenberg, L., Cattan, A., Schneider, M., Schlumberger, J. R., Amiel, J. L., Mathé, G.: La réanimation hématologique. I. Correction des troubles graves de la lignée érythrocytaire et des désorders de la coagulation. Presse méd. **74**, 769 (1966).

— — — — — — La réanimation hématologique. II. Correction des désorders graves des leucocytes et des immunoglobulins. La greffe de moelle osseuse. Presse méd. **74**, 1611 (1966).

— — — — — — Traitement symptomatique de l'agranulocytose par les transfusions de globules blancs. Presse méd. **74**, 1057 (1966).

— Mathé, G., Amiel, J. L., Cattan, A., Schneider, M., Schlumberger, J. R.: Adoptive immunotherapy by transfusions of leucocytes. Lancet **2**, 365 (1966).

— — De Grouchy, J., De Nava, C., De Vries, M. J., Amiel, J. L., Cattan, A., Schneider, M., Schlumberger, J. R.: White blood cell transfusions. Israel J. Med. Sci. **1**, 925 (1965).

— — Hayat, M., De Vassal, F., Amiel, J. L., Cattan, A., Schneider, M., Schlumberger, J. R., Rosenfeld, C., Jasmin, C.: Essai de traitement des leucémies aigues par la cytosine-arabinoside selon la méthode de Skipper. Nouv. Rev. franç. Hémat. **9**, 199 (1969).

— — — — — — — — — — Une nouvelle combinaison de méthotrexate-acide folinique pour le traitement des cancers (leucémies aigues et tumeurs solides). Presse méd. **77**, 385 (1969).

— Schneider, M., Cattan, A., Amiel, J. L., Schlumberger, J. R., Mathé, G.: Le traitement des leucémies aigues par la méthyl-glyoxal-bis (guanylhydrazone) et son association avec la 2-hydroxystilbamidine. Sem. Hôp. Paris **42**, 2955 (1966).

— — Mathé, G., Amiel, J. L., Cattan, A., Schlumberger, J. R.: White cell transfusions in the curative treatment and the prevention of infection. Colloque sur les transfusions de globules blancs. Éd.: C.N.R.S. Paris. Paris 1969 (sous presse).

Selawry, O. S., Hananian, J., Wolman, I. J., Abir, E., Chevallier, L., Gourdeau, R., Denton, R., Gussof, B. D., Levy, R., Burget, O., Mills, S. D., Blom, J., Jones, B., Patterson, R. B., McIntyre, O. R., Haurani, F. I., Moon, J. H., Hoogstraten, B., Kung, F. H., Sheehe, P. R., Frei, E. III., Holland, J. F.: New treatment schedule with improved survival in childhood leukemia (Acute leukemia group B). J. Amer. Ass. **194**, 75 (1965).

— James, D.: Therapeutic index of methotrexate as related to dose schedule and route of administration in children with acute lymphocytic leukemia. Proc. Amer. Ass. Cancer Res. **6**, 57 (1965).

Séman, G.: Presence de particules d'aspect viral dans les cellules du sang leucémique. Rev. franç. Étud. clin. biol. **13**, 763 (1968).

— An electron microscopical search for virus particles in patients with leukemias and lymphomas. Cancer **22**, 1033 (1968).

Tan, C. T. C., Phoa, J., Lyman, M., Murphy, M. L., Dargeon, H. W., Burchenal, J. H.: Hematological remissions in acute leukemia with cytophosphamide. Blood **18**, 808 (1961).

Thomas, E. D., Lochte, H. L., Cannon, J. H., Sahler, O. D., Ferrebee, J. W.: Supralethal whole body irradiation and isologous marrow transplantation. J. clin. Invest. **38**, 1709 (1959).

Yu, K. P., Clarckson, B.: Comparative studies of cytosine arabinoside (CA) and 5-fluoro-2'-deoxyuridine (FUdr) in leukemia in man. Proc. Amer. Ass. Cancer Res. **7**, 78 (1966).

Active Immunotherapy in the Treatment of Leukemia and Other Malignant Diseases in Animals and Man

G. Hamilton Fairley, D. Crowther, J. G. Guyer, R. M. Hardisty, H. E. M. Kay, P. J. Knapton, T. J. McElwain, and I. B. Parr

Institute of Cancer Research, Royal Marsden Hospital, and Hospital for Sick Children, Belmont, Sutton

With 2 Figures

I. Non-Specific Immunisation

It has been known for many years that various agents including oleic acid, BCG, and zymosan, which are capable of causing hyperplasia of the reticulo-endothelial system, also have the effect of retarding the growth of some tumours as well as accelerating homograft rejection (Murphy, 1924; Old et al., 1961; Weiss et al., 1961). Subsequently Halpern et al. (1963) and Smith and Woodruff (1968) showed a similar effect with Corynebacterium parvum.

Because of this work in animals and the results obtained by Mathé et al. (1968) using BCG to prolong remissions in acute lymphoblastic leukaemia, we decided to try the effect of another antigen (Bordetella pertussis) under similar circumstances, because this vaccine is known to produce a marked lymphocytosis in animals.

16 patients with acute lymphoblastic leukaemia in remission were divided into two groups, matched for age and sex. One group received regular injections of Bordetella pertussis, and the other had no treatment. The clinical findings in the two groups were similar with signs of systemic disease (lymphadenopathy, splenomegaly, etc.) in three of the controls and two of the test patients, and high peripheral blast counts (over 10,000/mm^3) in two cases in each group.

All the patients were in their first remission. In each group there were six patients in whom remissions had been obtained using prednisolone and vincristine, and in two by prednisolone and 6-mercaptopurine. Intensive "cyto-reductive" chemotherapy was given to all patients immediately following the induction of a complete remission. This consisted of five courses lasting five days each of 6-mercaptopurine and methotrexate in the patients already treated with vincristine; those who had already been given 6-mercaptopurine were also treated with cyclophosphamide. The period between each course varied depending on the degree of marrow suppression, but in all cases the intensive treatment was completed in a period of three months, and all patients were still in remission at the end of this therapy. The length of remission was measured from the last day of intensive chemotherapy.

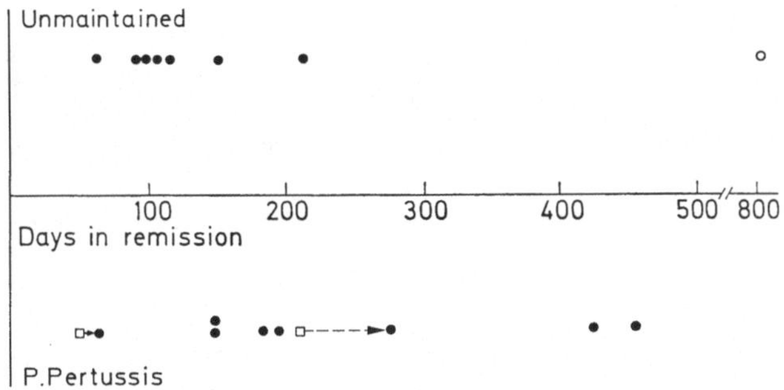

Fig. 1. The duration of first remission in patients either with no maintenance treatment or treated with Bordetella pertussis. Each circle represents an individual patient. ● Haematological relapse. □ Non-haematological relapse (first patient had meningeal leukaemia, and the second testicular involvement). ○ Still in remission

Half the patients were then treated with injections of Bordetella pertussis vaccine, either weekly or twice weekly by intramuscular injection given in a rotating system to the four quadrants of the body. The control group received no further therapy.

Follow-up on the two groups was the same. Total blood counts with white cell concentrates were examined every four weeks, and bone marrow aspirations performed every eight weeks. The results are shown in Fig. 1. Of the sixteen patients, all, except one control case, relapsed and were promptly brought into remission again by conventional means. Of the patients on pertussis vaccine one developed meningeal leukaemia, and another a testicular tumour prior to hematological relapse. In both these cases vaccination was continued during the treatment for the complication. During the extensive exposure to pertussis vaccine no child suffered any complications attributable to the vaccine.

The results are not impressive. There was a suggestion during the first 150 days that the duration of remission was being prolonged by immunisation with Bordetella pertussis, but this proved not to be the case. All the patients receiving immunotherapy have now relapsed, and the duration of remission is not comparable with that reported by Dr. JAMES HOLLAND using twice-weekly methotrexate. Subsequent work on the L5178Y lymphoma in mice in our laboratories has also shown that, in contrast to BCG, Bordetella pertussis has no protective effect on this tumour. We have, therefore, abandoned this method of immunisation.

We have now changed to using BCG, by a slightly different technique to that of MATHÉ et al. (1968). So far the results have not been encouraging, because we have been using this in patients who, although in remission, have had many relapses in the past. Our results merely confirm MATHÉ et al. (1968) that if immunotherapy is to be of any value it should only be given to patients with the minimal quantity of malignant disease (HAMILTON FAIRLEY, 1969).

II. Specific Immunisation

As yet we have not used irradiated leukaemic cells in the same way as MATHÉ et al. (1968) in man, but we have studied this method of immunisation in mice using the L5178Y lymphoma. It is quite easy in experimental animals to show that the

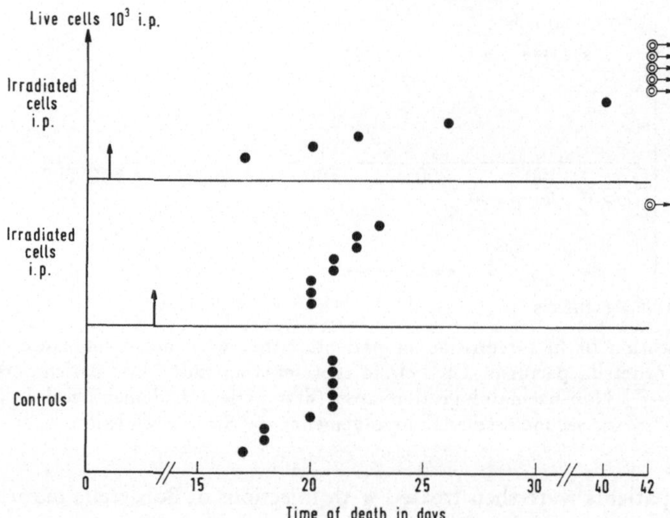

Fig. 2. The effect of immunising with irradiated lymphoma cells 24 hours and 3 days after the injection of 10^3 live lymphoma cells, using the L5178Y lymphoma in mice. Each circle represents an individual animal. ● Dead. ⊙→Alive and free from disease

injection of irradiated leukaemic cells will protect against a subsequent injection of live cells. However, it is much more important to demonstrate that immunisation with irradiated cells could have some effect on existing live leukaemic cells, because in human leukaemia even in remission many live cells are still present although they may not be detectable. Fig. 2 shows the survival of mice injected with 10^3 living malignant cells on Day 0, followed on Day 1 or Day 3 by 3×10^7 irradiated cells, both given by intraperitoneal injection. All the control animals had died by the 22nd day, but 5 out of 10 of the animals given irradiated cells 24 hours after live cells, and 1 out of 10 given irradiated cells 3 days later, survived free from disease for more than 42 days. Such results encourage one to pursue this form of immunotherapy in man, particularly in view of the results of Mathé et al. (1968) in acute lymphoblastic leukaemia.

A trial has now started between the Medical Research Council in Great Britain, and Professor Mathé's Department in Paris to test the effect of different forms of immunotherapy after intensive chemotherapy.

Summary

Following the work of Mathé showing that in patients with acute lymphoblastic leukaemia long remissions could be sustained by non-specific immunisation with BCG, we decided to try this form of treatment using Bordetella pertussis. The results were not impressive and certainly not comparable with the duration of remission obtainable by twice weekly methotrexate. We have now changed to using BCG and as yet it is too early to assess our results.

References

Halpern, B. N., Prevot, A. R., Biozzi, G., Stiffel, C., Mouton, D., Morard, J. C., Bouthillier, Y., Decreusefond, C.: Stimulation de l'activité phagocytaire du système réticulo-endothélial provoquée par Corynébacterium parvum. J. Reticulo-endothelial Soc. 1, 77 (1963).

Hamilton Fairley, G.: Immunity to malignant disease in man. Brit. med. J. **2**, 467 (1969).

Mathé, G., Amiel, J. L., Schwarzenberg, L., Schneider, M., Cattan, A., Schlumberger, J. R., Hayat, M., de Vassal, F.: Démonstration de l'efficacité de l'immunothérapie active dans la leucémie aigue lymphoblastique humaine. Rev. franç. Étud. clin. biol. **13**, 454 (1968).

Murphy, J. B.: The lymphocyte in resistance to tissue grafting, malignant disease and tuberculosis infection. An experimental study. Monogr. Rockefeller Inst. med. Res. **21** (1926).

Old, L. J., Benacerraf, B., Clarke, D. A., Carswell, E. A., Stockert, E.: The role of the reticulo-endothelial system in the host reaction to neoplasia. Cancer Res. **21**, 1281 (1961).

Smith, L. H., Woodruff, M. F. A.: Comparative effect of two strains of C. parvum on phagocytic activity and tumour growth. Nature (Lond.) **219**, 197 (1968).

Weiss, D. W., Bonhag, R. S., DeOrme, K. B.: Protective activity of fractions of tubercle bacilli against isologous tumours in mice. Nature (Lond.) **190**, 889 (1961).

III. Blastic Leukemias Secondary to Chronic Leukemias and Lymphomas

Therapy of the Blastic Phase of Chronic Granulocytic Leukemia

P. P. Carbone, G. P. Canellos, and V. T. De Vita

From the Medicine Branch, National Cancer Institute, National Institutes of Health, Bethesda, Maryland 20014

With 1 Figure

The accelerated or blastic phase of chronic granulocytic leukemia (CGL) ultimately leads to the demise of eighty percent of patients with this disease [1]. Anemia, thrombocytopenia, a rising percent of immature cells in the peripheral blood and bone marrow are the characteristic laboratory features. In addition some patients have moderate to extensive marrow fibrosis.

Clinically, fever, bone pain, and increasing fatigue are common complaints. On physical examination, massive splenomegaly is often present.

In addition to the Philadelphia chromosome other cytogenetic abnormalities such as aneuploidy and reduplication of the Philadelphia chromosome occur [2].

After the onset of blastic transformation, remission, with either reversion to the chronic phase or to a normal hematologic picture is rarely affected. Occasional remission, however, have been reported with the folic acid antagonist methotrexate [3] and the purine antagonist 6-mercaptopurine [4]. The survival of patients in the blastic phase of CGL has been invariably short, usually less than 3 months.

In the past several years fifty-six patients with chronic granulocytic leukemia in the blastic phase have been treated with six different treatment programs modeled after therapies used in patients with acute granulocytic leukemia. This report summarizes these results.

Patient Population

Fifty-six patients with chronic granulocytic leukemia in the accelerated phase have been treated between 1963 to the present time. The acute phase was defined as greater than forty percent abnormal myeloblasts in the bone marrow. In this report both Ph^1 positive and negative patients in the blast crisis are included.

Six additional patients in the chronic phase are included to illustrate the effect of a single dose of hydroxyurea on the peripheral blood cells.

The clinical trials were carried out in successive series and patients were allocated to the study in effect at the time. Because of the usually short survival, all but one patient remained on the same treatment program until his demise.

Treatment Programs

The treatment schedules, drug and initial dosages, are outlined in Tables 1—7. Modifications were made in doses for each patient individually to insure intensive treatment but a tolerable degree of toxicity. In general, those patients with marrow fibrosis at the onset of blast crisis, were more prone to the marrow suppressive effects of the drugs and ultimately more difficult to treat.

Supportive therapy in the form of red blood cell and platelet transfusions were usually necessary in all patients. Platelet transfusions were used for active bleeding and prophylactically for a platelet count less than 20,000/mm^3. White blood cells for transfusion were available from other patients in the chronic phase and were used for supportive purposes in the face of marrow aplasia associated with sepsis.

Definition of Response

A complete response (CR) was defined as a marrow with less than five percent myeloblasts, associated with a normal peripheral blood picture and no organomegally. An antileukemic effect (LE) less than a CR, was defined as a greater than fifty percent decrease in marrow and/or circulating myeloblasts and a decrease in organ size.

Results

Hydroxyurea (NSC 32065)

Hydroxyurea (HU) was given to 6 patients in 8 courses at a dose of 122—160 mg/kg in a single infusion over a 4 to 5 hour period (Table 1) [5]. The median fall in the white count was 55% occurring on the 4th to the 6th day. The absolute

Table 1. *Single dose hydroxyurea in CGL*

No. courses	Dose mg/kg	Initial WBC/mm^3	Percent fall WBC	Day of WBC nadir
8	130 [a] (122—160)	188 (119—250)	55 (43—64)	4 (4—6)

Mature PMN/mm$^3\times 10^3$ pre HU	Mature PMN/mm$^3\times 10^3$ post HU	Immature PMN [b]/mm$^3\times 10^3$ pre HU	Immature PMN/mm$^3\times 10^3$ post HU
116 (79.7—152.5)	60.6 (21—113)	65.5 (33.3—97.5)	6.7 (4.3—9.6)

[a] Median (range).

[b] Polymorphonuclear cell earlier than metamyclocytes.

granulocyte count fell to approximately one-half the pretreatment level whereas the absolute immature granulocytes (metamyelocytes, myelocytes and myeloblasts) dropped to 10.2% of the original level. This relatively dramatic and selective effect of HU on immature cells has been used repeatedly for rapid white blood cell lysis in patients with WBC counts in excess of 100,000 mm^3 and a high percentage of circulating peripheral blasts. Doses of 50 to 75 mg/kg for 1 to 3 days have been used prior to or in conjunction with the other treatment programs described here.

In 5 patients with CGL blastic crisis, hydroxyurea was given at doses of 15 to 100 mg/kg/day for 10 to 41 days (Table 2) [6]. In all patients, the white blood cell count and the abnormal cells in the peripheral blood declined and the spleen decreased in size. In 3 patients, the white blood cell count and the abnormal cells in the peripheral blood declined and the spleen decreased in size. In 3 patients severe pancytopenia ensued and death occurred in 10 to 41 days without a clinical remission.

Table 2. *Treatment CGL blastic crisis: hydroxyurea (NSC 32065)*

Dosages	Duration	No. patients
15—100 mg/kg/day	10—41 days	5

Response	Survival from onset treatment
CR – 0 LE – 5	10—41 days

Arabinosylcytosine (NSC 63878, Ara C)

Nine patients received Ara C at one of two schedules and dosages as outlined in Table 3. The median duration of treatment was 90 days (range 7—90 days). One patient achieved a complete remission that persisted for 8 months; the remission once obtained was maintained with 6-mercaptopurine. The median duration of survival in the group thus tested was 3 months.

Table 3. *Treatment CGL blastic crisis: arabinosyl cytosine (NSC 63878)*

Dosages	Duration of treatment	No. patients
30 mg/m^2 daily 100—200 mg/m^2 BIW	90 days (7—90)	9

Response	Survival from onset of treatment (months) [a]
CR – 1 LE – 4 NR – 4	1, 1, 2, 3, 3, 4, 7, 10 [b]

[a] One patient had other therapy for BC first.
[b] CR.

1,3 Bis (2-chlorethyl)-1-nitrosourea (NSC 409962, BCNU)

Four patients received BCNU as their primary treatment for the blastic crisis (Table 4). Two patients had marked reduction in circulating and bone marrow blasts at the height of toxicity but recovery was associated with return of blasts.

Table 4. *Treatment CGL blastic crisis: 1,3 bis (2-chlorethyl)-1-nitrosourea (BCNU) NSC 409962*

Dosage	No. courses	No. patients
125 mg/m²/day 3 day courses every 8 weeks	1 (1—2)	4

Response	Survival from onset treatment (months)
CR – 0 LE – 2 NR – 2	1/2, 1, 1, 3

BCNU and Ara C

Schabel and coworkers have reported "cell cures" of advanced L 1210 leukemia using a combination of these two agents on an every 4 hourly schedule for 24 hours repeated at 4 day intervals [7]. After a preliminary dose finding trials 13 patients received BCNU 40 mg/m² and Ara C 120 mg/m² in 24 hours divided over a twenty-four period in a six hourly schedule. This treatment was repeated every 4 days depending on toxicity for a median of 7 courses. One complete remission resulted in a patient following recovery from severe pancytopenia, and 3 patients had an anti-leukemic effect (Table 5).

As with the other treatments, death was caused by infection and/or hemorrhage in most patients. The median survival was 2 1/2 months. The patient who achieved complete remission had the longest survival.

Table 5. *Treatment CGL blastic crisis: BCNU and arbinosyl cytosine*

Dosage	No. courses	No. patients
BCNU 40— 60 mg/m² ARA-C 120—250 mg/m² q 3 days	7 (3—14)	13

Response	Survival from onset of treatment (months)
CR – 1 LE – 3 NR – 9	1/2, 1, 1 1/2, 2, 2 1/2, 2 1/2, 2 1/2, 3, 3, 3, 5, 5 1/2, 9

POMP Therapy [8]

A combination of prednisone, vincristine, methotrexate and mercaptopurine (POMP) was utilized in 13 patients following the report by Henderson et al. [9]

Table 6. *Treatment CGL blastic crisis: POMP*

Dosages (daily for 5 days)	No. courses	No. patients
Methotrexate 7.5 mg/m^2 Mercaptopurine 600 mg/m^2 Prednisone 10,000 mg/m^2 Vincristine 2 mg/m^2	4 (1—8)	13

Response	Survival from onset of treatment (months)
CR – 1 LE – 3 NR – 9	0, 1, 1, 2, 2, 2, 3, 3, 3, 5, 6, 6, 9, 9

who initially described the treatment program as a highly effective therapy in patients with acute granulocytic leukemia. Only one complete remission was achieved and three patients had a significant antileukemic effect; there were four deaths attributed to the extreme toxicity associated with the use of this combination (Table 6).

Vincristine and Prednisone [10]

The combination of vincristine (VCR) and prednisone has been long recognized as an effective inducer of remission in patients with acute lymphocytic leukemia of childhood. After a patient with known Ph[1] positive CGL for 42 months presented to the Clinical Center in the acute blastic crisis with a marrow characteristic of acute stem cell leukemia, this combination was attempted. This patient responded very dramatically to VCR and prednisone with a prompt remission not only the first time but subsequently on 2 other occasions following relapses. A total of 12 patients have received this combination and 3 complete remissions have been achieved that have lasted a total of 3, 10, and 14+ months. The latter two patients have had 2 and 3 successful reinduction attempts repectively during this time. All three patients have had aneuploidy as part of their cytogenetic analyses and none had splenomegaly (Table 7).

The summary of the NIH experience with blastic crisis is shown in Table 8. Of the 56 patients treated with the various regimens 6 (10.7%) had complete remissions.

Table 7. *Treatment CGL blastic crisis: vincristine — prednisone*

Dosages		Duration therapy (weeks)	No. patients
vincristine prednisone	2 mg/m^2 100 mg/day	4 (2—10)	12

Response	Survival from onset treatment (months)
CR – 3 LE – 7 NR – 2	1, 1+, 1½, 2+, 2, 2, 2, 5, 5, 8, 13, 14+

Table 8. *NCl treatment CGL blastic crisis: 1961—1969*

Drug	CR	LE	NR	Total
Hydroxyurea	0	5	0	5
ARA-C	1	4	4	9
BCNU	0	2	2	4
BCNU-ARA C	1	3	9	13
POMP	1	3	9	13
VCR-PRED	3	7	2	12
Totals	6	24	26	56
Percent	10.7	42.9	46.4	100

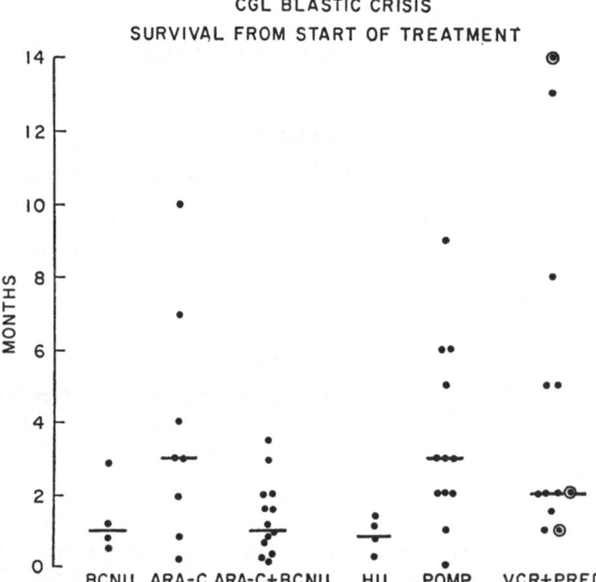

Fig. 1. Survival statistics for the various treatments for blastic crisis. Patients marked as ⊙ are still alive

Fig. 1 illustrates the comparative survival of all treatments. In only three of the programs were there survivals of any patients more than 6 months. The median survival varied between one and three months.

Discussion

The terminal phase of CGL resembles acute granulocytic leukemia (AGL) morphologically and similarly shares a low complete remission rate and short overall survival. While sporadic remissions have been reported in the acute phase of CGL no treatment program has resulted in 50% or more remissions as has been reported for AGL [9, 11]. In the present report treatment programs described as successful in

AGL such as Ara C [11] and POMP [9] have been used. Only with the latest program that of vincristine and prednisone was the number of complete remissions more than one in any treatment program. The advantage of this program has been its relative lack of severe myelosuppression. Daunomycin, another agent reported to be active against acute granulocytic leukemia has not as yet received adequate trial in the blastic phase of CGL [12].

It seems significant that in the present report remissions have been achieved only in those patients with aneuploid cell lines. During remission the cytogenetic analyses indicated a return to a single cell line with 46 chromosomes and the Ph^1 chromosome. Thus successful therapy designed to cure patients must not only return the hematologic state to normal but must eradicate the Ph^1 chromosome marrow cells. With modern techniques of tissue typing allogenic marrow transplantation may offer an alternative modality of therapy. THOMAS and coworkers have already utilized this method of therapy with a definite but temporary response [13]. The major obstacle to the successful use of this method is the control of the graft versus host reaction.

Summary

The accelerated or blastic phase of chronic granulocytic leukemia leads to the demise of 80 percent of patients with this disease. Fifty-six patients with acute phase of chronic granulocytic leukemia have been treated with a variety of chemotherapy programs. Complete responses were seen in 10.7 percent. The most effective program was the combination of vincristine and prednisone. The median survival from onset of blastic crisis was one to three months.

References

1. DAMESHEK, W., GUNZ, F.: In: Leukemia. Ed.: GRUNE & STRATTON. New York 1964, p. 223.
2. WHANG PENG, J., CANELLOS, G. P., CARBONE, P. P.: Clinical implications of cytogenic variants in chronic myelogenous leukemia (CML). Blood **32,** 755—766 (1968).
3. HUGULEY, C. M., JR., VOGLER, W. R., LEA, J. W., CORLEY, C. C., JR., LOWERY, M. E.: Acute leukemia treated with divided doses of methotrexate. Arch. int. Méd. exp. **115,** 23—28 (1965).
4. ELLISON, R. R., BURCHENAL, J. H.: Treatment of chronic granulocytic leukemia with the 6 substituted purines 6 mercaptopurine thioguanine and 6 chlorpurine. Clin. Pharmacol. Ther. **1,** 631—644 (1960).
5. FISHBEIN, W.: Excretion and hematologic effects of single intravenous infusion in patients with chronic myeloid leukemia. Johns Hopk. med. J. **121,** 1—8 (1967).
6. FISHBEIN, W. N., CARBONE, P. P., FREIREICH, E. J., MISRA, P., FREI, E. III: Clinical trials of hydroxyurea in patients with cancer and leukemia. Clin. Pharmacol. Ther. **5,** 574 to 580 (1964).
7. SCHABEL, F. M., JR.: Relationship of cell population kinetics and therapy. In: The prolification and spread of neoplastic cells. Baltimore: The Williams & Wilkins Company 1968.
8. FOLEY, H. T., BENNETT, J. M.: CARBONE, P. P.: Combination chemotherapy in accelerated phase of chronic granulocytic leukemia. Arch. int. Méd. exp. **123,** 166—170 (1969).
9. HENDERSON, E. S., SERPICK, A.: Effect of combination drug therapy and prophylactic oral antibiotic treatment in adult acute leukemia. Clin. Res. **15,** 336 (1967).
10. CANELLOS, G. P., WHANG-PENG, J.: Effect of vincristine in blastic transformation of chronic granulocytic leukemia: cytogenetic correlation. Clin. Res. **17,** 400 (1969).
11. HENDERSON, E., SERPICK, A., LEVENTHAL, B., HENRY, P.: Cytosine arabinoside infusions in adult and childhood acute myelocytic leukemia. Proc. Amer. Ass. Cancer Res. **9,** 29 (1968).
12. BERNARD, J., BOIRON, M., JACQUILLAT, C., WEIL, M.: Rubidomycin in 400 patients with leukemia and other malignancies. Abst. Simult. Sessions 12th Cong. Int. Soc. Hemat. **5** (1968).
13. THOMAS, D., BUCKNER, D.: Personal communication.

Blastic Crisis in Chronic Leukemia and Polycythemia vera

J. Bousser, G. Bilski-Pasquier, J. Briere, and F. Reyes

Hôpital de l'Hôtel-Dieu, Paris

With 1 Figure

One hundred cases of chronic granulocyte leukemia and 150 cases of polycythemia vera were rewieved. We report here 22 cases of blastic crisis in chronic C. M. L. and 3 cases in polycythemia vera.

The first difficulty in the appreciation of the effects of treatment is a good definition of blastic crisis. Our definition is the following one: a blastic or promyelocytic involvement of blood, bone marrow or glandular nodes, isolated or together with a percentage greater than 25 to 30 immature cells. Others definitions near enough may be given recording J. Bernard [1], P. Carbone [2], Morrow [3], J. Debray [4]. The Karanas' criteria [5] are more complex and concerned the terminal phase sooner than the blastic crisis. The second difficulty is to catch easily the very just time of incipient blastic crisis in the course of chronic phase. Its onset's time is extremely variable.

In our short serie the mediane is 18 months [1]. Range is very wide less than 3 to more 90 months (Fig. 1). Its early or delayed nature is hardly expected and often doubtfull. For running signs are scattered in time and miscellaneous (fever, weakness, involvement of bones, lymph nodes in largement, anemia, thrombopenia, basophilic granulocytes, transient blastic cells in blood). Waiting for a number of 30% of immature cells lead to a too late diagnosis and treatment. Even after an increase of the total immaturity count over 30%, clinical and hematological picture will be not necessarily clear cut.

Cytological and cytochemical data are moreover various: myeloblastic, lymphoblastic, undifferentiated, miscellaneous and once we have observed a double population. Nevertheless we remain faithfull to our definition, i. e., 30% of immature cells. In these conditions we undertook three trials of treatment with one, or two, or three simultaneous drugs (Table 1).

In the 3 cases of polycythemia vera the patients dead very quickly, before an effective treatment.

In conclusion, in that short serie the results are poor. Two explanations are available: 1) the heavier toxicity of drugs on a bone marrow previously injured by

[1] In an other serie of 94 cases, J. Briere observed a mediane of 25 months. In our serie a selective effect explains the difference of 7 months.

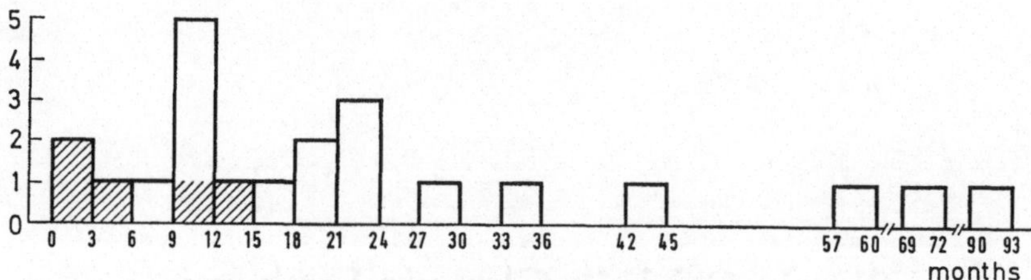

Dibromomannitol; □ Busulfan

Fig. 1. Time of blastic crisis onset related with the treatment of chronic phase

Table 1

	Number of course	Total failure	Partial remission	Complete remission
Prednisone (2 mg/kg)	1	1		
6 M.P. (2.5 mg/kg)	1	1		
Methyl GAG (200 to 300 mg/m², 2 to 3 time a week)	2	1	1	
Prednisone and Methyl GAG	4	2	1	1
Methyl GAG and 6 M.P.	4	2	2	
Prednisone and Methotrexate	1	1		
Prednisone and 6 M.P.	7	3	4	
Methyl GAG 6 M.P. Prednisone	7	6	1	
Methyl GAG Prednisolone Rubidomycine (1 mg/kg)	2	1		1

Results (summarrized)

Total number of patients: 25 (22 C M L, 3 polycythemia vera)
Total number of courses of treatment: 29
Total failure: 18
Incomplete remission: 9
Complete remission: 2

a long chronic phase and its treatment; 2) the delayed diagnosis allowing an extensive proliferation of immature cells. We hope so to obtain a better definition of blastic crisis and perhaps to have a preventive treatment by using, already in chronic phase, drugs know to be effective on acute phase, in iteratives cures, like for instance, corticotherapy as proposed G. MATHÉ.

References

1. BERNARD, J., SELIGMAN, M., KVICALA, R.: La transformation aigue de la leucémie myéloïde chronique. Rev. franç. Étud. clin. biol. 4, 1024 (1959).
2. FOLEY, H. T., BENNETT, J. M., CARBONE, P.: Combination chemotherapy in accelerated phase of chronic myelocytic leukemia. Arch. int. Méd. exp. 123, 166 (1969).
3. MORROW, G., PEASE, G., STROEBEL, C., BENNETT, J. M.: Terminal phase of chronic myelogenous leukemia. Cancer 18, 369 (1965).
4. DEBRAY, J.: La transformation aigue de la leucémie myéloïde chronique. Colloque sur les aspects actuels de la leucémie myéloïde (G. MARCHAL). Sem. Hôp. Paris 36, 46 (1959).
5. KARANAS, A., SILVER, R.: Characteristics of the terminal phase of chronic granulocytic leukemia. Blood 32, 3 (1968).
6. BRIERE, J.: Contribution à l'étude des leucémies myéloïdes à chromosome Philadelphie, d'évolution rapide. Thèse. Paris 1969.

Treatment of Blastic Crisis in Chronic Myelocytic Leukemia

A. Cattan, G. Mathé, J. L. Amiel, J. R. Schlumberger, L. Schwarzenberg, M. Schneider, and L. Berumen

Institut de Cancérologie et d'Immunogénétique, Hôpital Paul-Brousse, 14, avenue Paul-Vaillant Couturier et Institut Gustave Roussy, 16, avenue Paul-Vaillant Couturier, 94-Villejuif, France

The development of an acute leukaemic syndrome can perhaps be considered to be the usual evolution of chronic myeloid leukaemia. Its occurrence is feared and its prognosis is still very poor, despite recent advances in treatment. Twenty-nine patients have been studied, 14 males and 15 females, their ages were 16—71 years (median 40 years). The acute leukaemic syndrome appeared 3 weeks to 7 years after the apparent onset of chronic myeloid leukaemia (median 26 months).

During the course of the chronic myelocytic leukaemia, 21 patients were treated by chemotherapy, one given splenic irradiation, 4 given a combination of chemotherapy and splenic irradiation at different phases of the disease, and 3 were untreated. Five of the patients treated by chemotherapy were subjected to systematic splenectomy, with the intention of both helping to eradicate the leukaemia and preventing the disorders caused by splenomegaly in the advanced stage of the disease. The splenectomy was carried out during a period of remission.

Since the acute leukaemic syndrome was seen not only after radiotherapy but also after chemotherapy, it does not appear to be solely the consequence of radiotherapy. Systematic splenectomy did not prevent the acute leukaemic transformation but perhaps delayed its time of onset. The average duration of chronic myeloid leukaemia before the appearance of the acute leukaemic syndrome was 21 months in 21 patients without splenectomy and 42 months in 5 patients treated by systematic splenectomy. However, there is no statistically significant difference between these two groups, as there are too few patients in the second group.

The acute leukaemic syndrome was heralded by fever (8 patients), bone pain (4 patients), a haemorrhagic syndrome (4 patients), the appearance of blast cells in the circulating blood (9 patients). Sometimes these events occurred 2 to 3 months before the diagnosis could be confirmed by examination of the bone marrow. More than 15 per cent of blast cells in at least one sector of the bone marrow was considered to be significant of an acute leukaemic transformation; this was always confirmed by a second marrow examination 15 days to 1 month later. The prognosis was very grave; survival was 1 week to 15 months, with a median survival of 1.5 months.

Table 1. *Results of treatment of blastic crisis in chronic myelocytic leukaemia*

Treatment	No. of courses	Remissions		Failures	
		Complete	Partial	Partial	Total
Prednisone	4	1	1		2
Vincristine	10	3	1	1	5
Methyl-hydrazine-bis(guanylhydrazone)	16	2	1	1	12
Methyl-GAG + 2-hydroxystilbamidine	1				1
Cytosine-arabinoside	1				1
Methotrexate + folinic acid	3		1		2
L-asparaginase	1				1
Prednisone + vincristine + rubidomycine	1		1		
+ methyl-GAG	4	1	1		2
+ L-asparaginase	4		1	1	2
+ cytosine arabinoside	1			1	
Prednisone + rubidomycine + methyl-GAG + cytosine arabinoside	1				1
Total	47	7	7	4	29

Table 1 summarises the different drugs used in our patients and their results. Out of 47 courses of therapy, 14 remissions were obtained, of which 3 occurred in the same patient, 2 in 2 patients and 1 in 7 patients. Nineteen patients failed to obtain any remission. Among the drugs used, the best results appeared to be obtained with vincristine (remissions in 4 out of 10 patients) and prednisone (remissions in 2 out of 4 patients). The recent combinations of various drugs (methotrexate and folinic acid; prednisone and vincristine and rubidomycin these three drugs plus methyl-gag or plus asparaginase, or + cytosine arabinoside prednisone + rubidomycin + methyl-gag + cytosine arabinoside), did not appear to be followed by satisfactory results (1 complete remission, 4 incomplete remissions, out of 14 courses of therapy).

In 4 patients, the disappearance of the blast cells from the marrow was accompanied by the reappearance of the picture of chronic myeloid leukaemia.

Various complications were seen during the development of the acute leukaemic syndrome (Table 2). Disorders of haemostasis were observed in 22 patients; 10 had a haemorrhagic diathesis, most often as the result of thrombocytopenia. This sometimes preceded the acute leukaemic transformation and was not constant during its course. Thrombosis or diffuse intravascular coagulation were seen in 6 patients; and on six occasions there was a combination of haemorrhage and thrombosis. These complications led to the death of four patients. The picture most commonly seen, despite all other biochemical disturbances, was a marked reduction in the level of factors II, V, VII and X, without a notable change in the level of fibrinogen nor of the values of overall tests of coagulation. A severe infection supervened in 18 patients; in 3 of them it was fatal, and it was often accompanied by disorders of haemostasis. This combination caused the death of 9 patients. In 4 cases of aplasia, only one was fatal, due to a syndrome of haemorrhage and infection; a perforating gastric ulcer occurred in 4 patients, in one of them it was associated with a perforation of the small in-

Table 2. *Complications observed during the development of acute leukaemic syndrome*

Disorders of hemostasis	Haemorrhage	10	22
	Intravascular coagulation	6	
	Both	6	
Infections	Septicemia	2	18
	Staphylococcia	4	
	Mycosis (aspergillus, mucor)	2	
	Fever	7	
	Others (zona, herpes, icterus)	3	
Aplasia			4
Gastric ulcer (perforated)			4
Small bowel perforation			1
Myocarditis			2

Table 3. *Causes of death*

Marrow aplasia		1
Disorders of haemostasis	Thrombosis and/or intravascular coagulation	2
	Haemorrhage	2
Infection		3
Infection and disorders of hemostasis		9
Perforating ulcer (stomach or intestinal)		4
Myocarditis		2
Various		4
Not defined		2

Table 4. *Efficiency of treatment according to the morphology of blast cells*

Cell appearance	No. of patients	Effect of treatment: Complete remissions	Partial remissions
Lymphoblast like	10	5	0
Myeloblast like	9	0	1
Mixed	10	2	6

testine, all of which were fatal. In 2 patients, death resulted from a toxic myocarditis caused by rubidomycin (Table 3).

It seems likely that the efficiency of treatment is partly related to the morphology of the blast cells. In 10 patients the cells, when stained conventionally, looked like lymphoblasts, and in 10 others the morphology was mixed, some cells looking like lymphoblasts and others like myeloblasts. Five complete remission were observed in the first group, whilst only a single, incomplete remission was obtained in the second group. The results in the third group fell between the other two groups (Table 4).

Discussion

An acute leukaemic syndrome is sufficiently frequent during the evolution of chronic myeloid leukaemia to be thought of as the natural termination of this disease. It accounted for 75 per cent of the deaths in chronic myeloid leukaemia in 1959 [1], and in our own patients it is greater than 90 per cent. The acute leukaemia is not uniquely related to previous radiotherapy; splenectomy does not stop its occurrence, though it perhaps retards its progress.

The prognosis of this syndrome is very poor, despite modern therapy complete remissions can only be achieved in 10 to 15 per cent of the patients and their median survival is short. The cytological appearances of the blast cells seems to be of some value when assessing the prognosis.

References

1. Bernard, J., Seligmann, M., Kvicala, R.: La transformation aigüe de la leucémie myéloïde chronique. Rev. franç. Étud. clin. biol. 10, 1024 (1959).
2. Mathé, G., Seman, G.: Aspects histologiques et cytologiques des leucémies et hémato-sarcomes, Vol. 1. Ed.: Maloine. Paris 1963.
3. — Tubiana, M., Calman, F., Schlumberger, J. R., Berumen, L., Choquet, C., Cattan, A., Schneider, M.: Les syndromes de leucémie aigüe (SLA) apparaissant au cours de l'évolution des hématosarcomes et des leucémies chroniques (Analyse clinique). Nouv. Rev. franç. Hémat. 7, 543 (1967).
4. Strumia, M. M., Strumia, P. V., Bassert, D.: Splenectomy in leukemia: hematologic and clinical effects on 34 patients and review of 299 published cases. Cancer Res. 26, 519 (1966).
5. Tivey, H.: The prognosis for survival in chronic granulocytic and lymphocytic leukemia. Amer. J. Roentgenol. 72, 68 (1954).

Cell Proliferation in Chronic Myeloid Leukemia under Discontinuous Treatment from Diagnosis to Blastic Crisis

P. A. Stryckmans, J. Manaster, T. Peltzer, M. Socquet, and G. Vamecq

Department of Internal Medicine, Institut Jules Bordet, University of Brussels

With 8 Figures

There are no methods available presently to study the growth of the whole body pool of immature myeloid cells in chronic myeloid leukemia (CML). It is evident, from clinical observation, that this pool is greatly increased in CML, that it can be considerably reduced repeatedly by specific treatments and that it can regrow after cessation of therapy. Moxley and coworkers [1] and Galbraith [2] have shown that immature myeloid cells in the blood are exchanging rapidly with marrow and spleen immature myeloid cells. Vincent and coworkers [3] have shown that the labeling indices of myelocytes after in vivo or in vitro incubation with tritiated thymidine are similar in the blood and in the bone marrow of these patients and that the time for DNA synthesis is similar in blood and bone marrow (BM).

Fig. 1 represents a model based on these concepts. The central box represents the blood compartment. It is composed of mature granulocytes and immature myeloid cells. The mature cells appear to be the end product of the immature cells from the BM, the spleen and the blood. The immature cells of the blood on the other hand do not represent an end product of the proliferating compartments but represent rather a fraction of the whole proliferating pool. It was considered therefore that the growth of the total pool of myeloid precursors could be studied by the observation of the growth of its circulating fraction i. e. the immature cells of the blood which are easily accessible for multiple sampling.

In a retrospective study, 13 patients were selected from a group of patients with CML treated in our Institute in the past 15 years. The selection was made on the following basis: (1) that the patients were treated by at least 2 consecutive courses of myleran and/or ^{32}P. (2) that the treatment was given intermittently without maintenance therapy during the period of observation. The absolute numbers of circulating myeloblasts (M_1), promyelocytes (M_2), myelocytes (M_3 and M_4) and metamyelocytes (M_5), in the blood were added together. These cells were considered as one single compartment of circulating immature myeloid cells (CIMC). This compartment always decreased in an exponential fashion, as a consequence of the treatment. After cessation of therapy, it always started to increase in an exponential

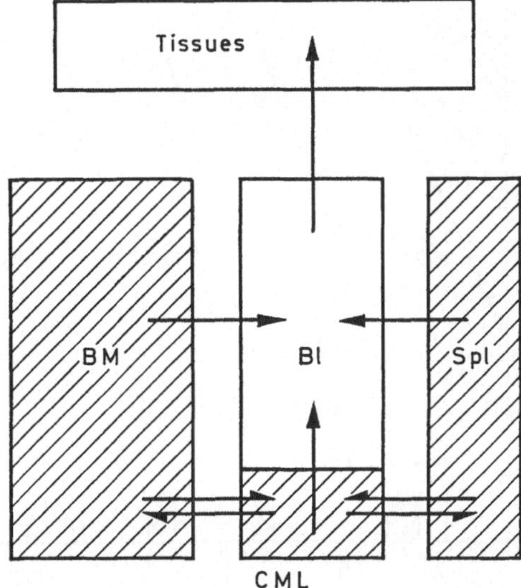

Fig. 1. Stippled rectangles represent different compartments of immature myeloid cells. The white rectangles represent mature granulocytes. BM: bone marrow, BL: blood, Spl: spleen

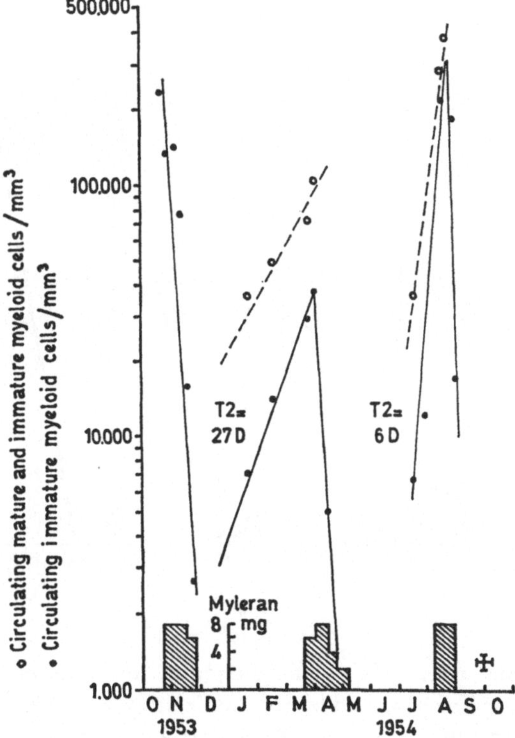

Fig. 2. o Circulating mature and immature myeloid cells/mm^3. ● Circulating immature myeloid cells/mm^3

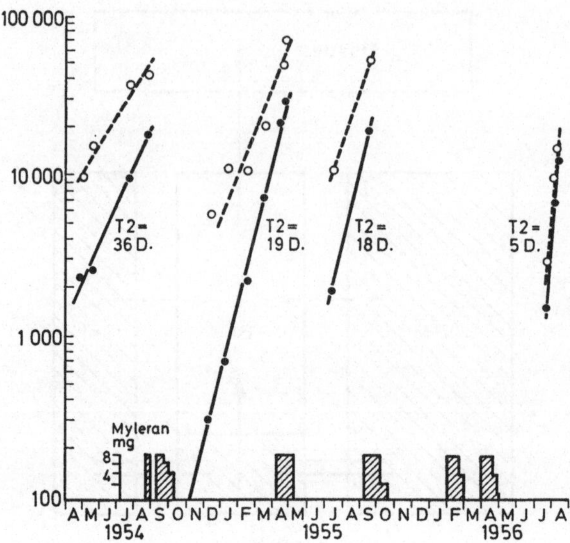

Fig. 3. o Circulating mature and immature myeloid cells/mm³. ● Circulating immature myeloid cells/mm³

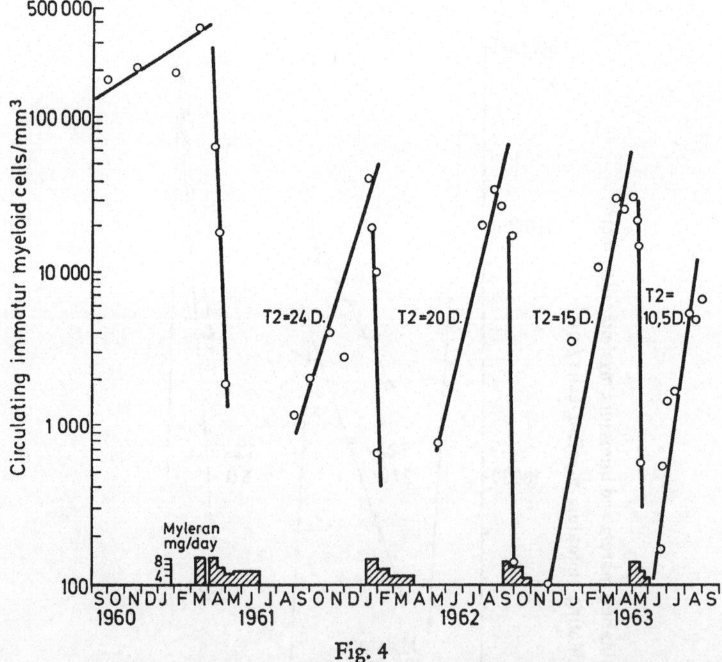

Fig. 4

fashion. The doubling time (T_2) of the immature myeloid cells was measured at intervals from the base line procured by the administration of treatment.

Fig. 2 shows on semilog paper the linear increase of circulating immature myeloid cells represented by the solid line. The first ascending solid line shows a doubling time (indicated as T_2) of 27 days, whereas the second increase observed after a

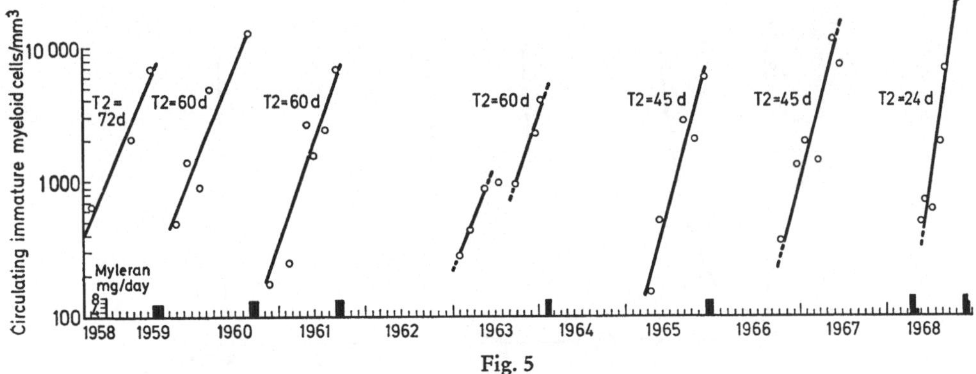

Fig. 5

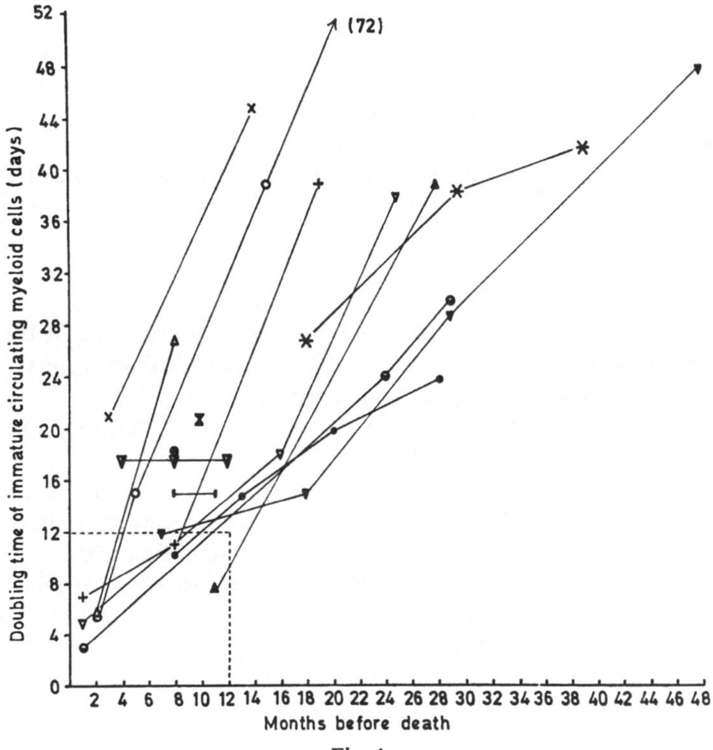

Fig. 6

second course of myleran, during the blastic crisis has a T_2 of 6 days. It thus shows an acceleration of the doubling time from one period to the next.

Fig. 3 shows four consecutive increases of circulating immature myeloid cells: the first with a T_2 of 36 days; the second, 19 days; the fourth before death represents the blast crisis with a T_2 of 5 days.

Fig. 4 shows 5 consecutive increases of blood immature myeloid cells over a period of 3 years. The 5th does not represent the blast crisis yet. The patient died 6 months later in blast crisis.

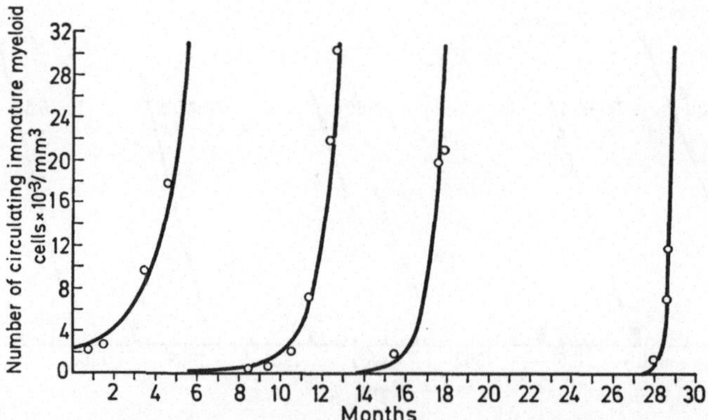

Fig. 7. o Observed values, — computed values

Fig. 5 shows the evolution of the disease of a patient who is still alive more than 10 years after the diagnosis of her disease. She was treated by myleran only. The successive increases become steeper with the years.

Fig. 6 summarizes the results of the 12 patients who died. In ordinate is shown the doubling time of the blood immature myeloid cells and in abcissa the time when T_2 was observed in months prior to the moment of death. A different symbol is used for each patient and each line joins the successive estimates of T_2 made on one particular patient. It is shown that 2 patients showed no progressive shortening of the doubling time of the circulating myeloid cells. It is also shown that the 9 cases in which T_2 decreased below 12 days died within the year. A short T_2 may, therefore, be considered as a sign announcing the blast crisis.

The first question that arises is whether the decrease of T_2 with time might reflect progressive resistance to treatment. Actually, the half time of the CIMC as a consequence of the treatment was always of the order of 6 days and did not change significantly during the evolution of the disease. This seems to indicate that the effect of the treatment on cells was unchanged in this series of patients.

The second question that arises is whether the progressive shortening of T_2 is either the result of successive changes occuring step by step, discontinuously, as a consequence of each course of treatment or rather a continuous phenomenon representing the natural evolution of the disease. A mathematical model was considered in which an exponential growth would itself accelerate continuously in an exponential fashion [1].

On Fig. 7 the solid lines represent the computed values of such a continuously accelerating phenomenon which has to be reset however to lower values after each course of treatment. The observed values are represented by the black circles. They fit fairly with the theoretical values. This does not prove but supports the hypothesis that the observed acceleration is continuous and therefore independent of treatment.

---

[1] More explicitly the function is of the form $N = pe^{qe^{rt}}$ in which N: the number of circulating immature myeloid cells at time t. p: a parameter readjusted for each growth between two successive treatments. q and r: parameters constant for each particular patient under study.

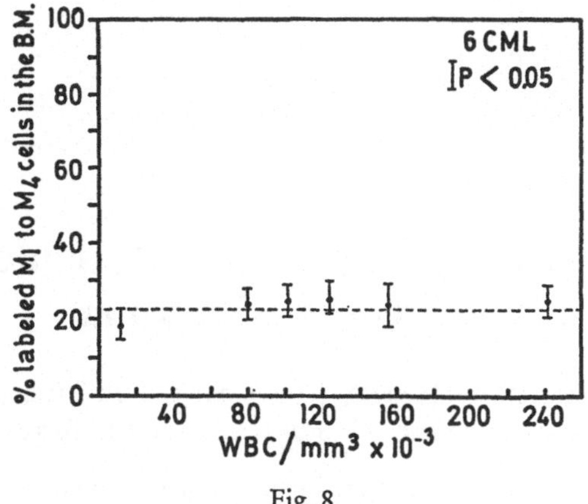

Fig. 8

The third question that arises is whether the shortening of the doubling time could be a reflexion of a shortening of the generation time. The LI of the myeloid precursors (M_1 to M_4) in the BM *of 6 CML patients* was determined after in vitro incubation of the BM with ^{3}HT dr. Fig. 8 shows that these LI in the BM patients at different moments of the evolution of their disease were not significantly different. No significant correlation was found either between the LI of the BM myeloid precursors and the number of leucocytes in the blood.

In conclusion, the increase of immature myeloid cells in the blood is getting faster and faster up to the moment of the blast crisis. This could represent the natural evolution of the disease independent of treatments. Nothing indicates that this is the result of an accelerated proliferation of the recognizable myeloid cells. It is suggested that the defect is probably located at the level of the unrecognizable stem cell.

Summary

Fourteen patients with CML, treated with Myleran and/or ^{32}P intermittently for several years till the blastic transformation, were studied retrospectively. The absolute number of circulating immature myeloid cells (CIMC) was determined at regular intervals. Between two successive courses of treatment, the increase of the CIMC was exponential. The doubling time of the successive increases in 12 patients became progressively shorter. It is suggested that this growth of the CIMC is a reflexion of the growth of the total pool of immature myeloid cells in the body. There was no evidence for a progressive resistance to the treatment. In a prospective study of 6 patients with CML no indication was found for a progressive shortening of the generation time of the recognizable immature myeloid cells.

References

1. Moxley, J. H., Perry, S., Weiss, G. H., Zelen, M.: Return of leucocytes to the bone marrow in chronic myelogenous leukaemia. Nature **208**, 1281 (1965).
2. Galbraith, P. R.: Studies on the longevity, sequestration and release of the leukocytes in chronic myelogenous leukemia. Canad. med. Ass. J. **95**, 511 (1966).
3. Vincent, P. C., Cronkite, E. P., Greenberg, M. L., Kirsten, C., Schiffer, L. M., Stryckmans, P. A.: Leukocyte kinetics in chronic myeloid leukemia. I. DNA synthesis time in blood and marrow myelocytes. Blood **33**, 843 (1969).

Blastic Leukemia Complicating Reticulo-Sarcoma and Lympho-Sarcoma

J. R. SCHLUMBERGER, G. MATHÉ, J.-L. TEXIER, J. L. AMIEL, A. CATTAN, L. SCHWARZENBERG, M. SCHNEIDER, and L. BERUMEN

Institut de Cancérologie et d'Immunogénétique, Hôpital Paul-Brousse, 14, avenue Paul-Vaillant-Couturier, et Institut Gustave-Roussy, 16, avenue Paul-Vaillant-Couturier, 94-Villejuif, France

With 2 Figures

A blastic leukaemia may appear in the course of a malignant lymphoma (Table 1): it is exceptional in Hodgkin's disease, in follicular lymphoma, in reticulosarcoma, histiocytic type and in lymphosarcoma, lymphocytic type, but it is frequent in reticulosarcoma, histioblastic type (distinction between these two types of reticulosarcoma has been justified and illustrated by MATHÉ et al., 1967, 1970) and in lymphosarcoma, lymphoblastic type.

Table 1. *Acute leukaemia secondary to malignant lymphomas*

Malignant lymphomas	Number of cases studied	Number of leukaemia
Reticulosarcoma		
Histiocytic type	43	0
Histioblastic type	131	15
Lymphosarcoma		
Lymphocytic type	4	0
Lymphoblastic type	146	38
Lymphoma, follicular type	39	1
Hodgkin's disease	403	0

Reticulosarcoma (Histioblastic Type)

Since 1966, we have collected 15 cases of "histiomonoblastic" leukaemia appearing during the evolution of histioblastosarcoma.

The morphologic type of leukaemic cells is very similar to the one found in the usual case of acute monoblastic leukaemia: cytology, cytochemistry (esterases) did not allow us to differentiate any specific characteristics. So, it seems that this type of acute leukaemia may be qualified as histiomonoblastic.

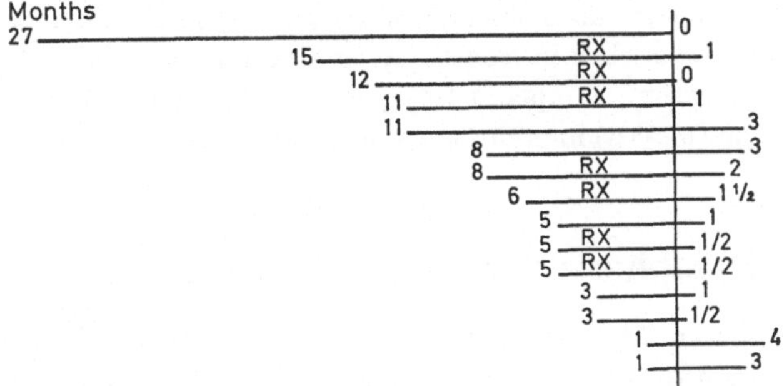

Fig. 1. Acute blastic (histiomonoblastic) leukaemia appearing in the course of reticulosarcoma (histioblastic type): duration of the disease before (on the left) and after (on the right) the appearance of the blastic leukemia

Fig. 1 shows that these blast cells, appear late in the course of the illness, in the bone marrow and in the blood; they are frequently accompanied by less differentiated blast cells [1].

The left part of the table shows the duration of the illness before manifestation of the acute leukaemia.

Once these manifestations appear, the prognosis is very poor: survival is less than 4 months after the onset of the leukaemia and averages about one month.

One notes that the whole duration of the disease is about the same in histioblastic and histiocytic types of these sarcomas, but, again histiomonoblastic leukaemia complicates only the histioblastic type.

In two of ours cases, the acute leukaemia appeared without any tumor recurrence.

Chemotherapeutic attempts to induce remissions are shown on the Table 2. Drug combinations (6th and 8th line) seem to produce the best results in the course of the illness, except for cytosine arabinoside, which seems to be able to be effective alone.

Table 2. *Results of chemotherapy in acute histio-monoblastic leukaemia secondary to reticulum cell sarcoma, histioblastic type*

Drugs	Remissions (weeks)		
	Complete	Partial	Failures
Prednisone	1 (4)	1 (12)	
Cytosine arabinoside	1 (4)		
Vincristine + prednisone	1 (4)		2 (3, 4)
Methotrexate + folinic acid	2 (2, 3)		1 (2)
Methyl-hydrazine + T.E.M. + prednisone	3 (4, 4, 4)	1 (12)	1 (3)
Vincristine + prednisone + L-asparaginase	1 (12)		
Methyl-hydrazine + prednisone + nitrogen mustard	1 (3)		
Methyl-hydrazine + T.E.M. + vinblastine + prednisone	1 (12)		1 (8)
Total	11 / 18	2 / 18	5 / 18

In these cases, the remissions observed were rare and so short that we have expressed them in *weeks* rather than in months. After a very severe clinical history, death is due, among other reasons, to aplasia (drug toxicity in 9 cases) as well as to severe hepatic dysfunction (6 cases) in addition to the fatal relapses.

Lymphosarcoma (Lymphoblastic Type)

We have also seen 20 new cases of acute lymphoblastic leukaemia since 1967 (Table 1) in addition to the 18 already published (MATHÉ, 1967). This makes a total of 38 cases. We eliminated 5 cases with lymphoblastic tumors of the mediastinum or of the abdomen. In these particular cases the bone marrow was positive within less than a week of the appearance of the initial symptomes. Such cases were conventionally classified as "leukosarcomatosis" and are nothing else but typical primary acute lymphoblastic leukaemias.

The frequency of this syndrome of leukaemic transformation of lymphoblastosarcomas is about 30% of the cases. We have seen this leukaemia always after the same type of malignant lymphoma: a malignant lymphoma defined as lymphoblastic lymphosarcoma. But we have never seen the acute leukaemic syndrome evolving out of lymphocytic lymphosarcoma, chronic lymphocytic leukaemia, etc.

The lymphoblastic cells appearing in the bone marrow during the leukaemic period, seem a little less differentiated than those that may be seen in the malignant tissue during the non leukaemic phase; in this phase the cells are more evocative of "prolymphocytes" (MATHÉ et al., 1967).

Systematic counting of blast cells in the circulating blood, "leucoconcentration technique" (i. e. presence of lymphoblasts in abnormally high concentration in the blood) allows earlier diagnosis of the leukaemic diffusion.

In Fig. 2 the left part shows the duration of the illness before the appearance of the leukaemia. The dotted lines on the right part of the figure represent the patients that are still alive.

The first case had several adenopathic manifestations treated by local radiotherapy. The second case had a long history of a nodular histologic type (Brill-Symmers).

Cases 1 and 3 had only a temporary presence of lymphoblasts in the bone marrow and blood; this seems to be of no significance since the prognosis was not any better than for the other cases.

Relapses in the form of isolated lymphoblastic meningitis (2 cases) gave a poor prognosis (partial remission of 4 months in 1 case, and death after 1 month in the second case).

We have attempted various chemotherapeutic trials to induce remission. Isolated drugs produce such poor results that associated drugs must be employed to induce remission. These must then be followed by complementary therapy (Table 3).

These treatments do lead to some long lasting remissions; five of the 20 patients studied are still in complete remission.

To conclude, appearance of blastic leukaemia syndrome in these two kinds of malignant lymphomas (i. e. histioblastosarcomas and lymphoblastosarcomas) is relatively frequent: the leukaemic syndrome is more than two times more frequent after lymphoblastosarcoma than after histioblastosarcoma. Their prognosis is very bad after histioblastosarcoma, and little better after lymphoblastosarcoma.

New drug combinations must be tried to improve their prognosis.

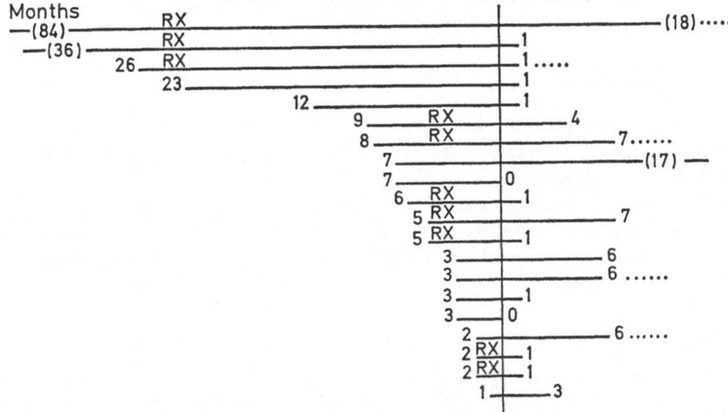

Fig. 2. Acute blastic (lymphoblastic) leukaemia appearing in the course of lymphosarcoma (lymphoblastic type): duration of the disease before (on the left) and after (on the right) the appearance of the blastic leukemia

Table 3. *Results of chemotherapy in lymphoblastic leukaemia secondary to lymphosarcomas, lymphoblastic type*

Drugs	Remissions (months) Complete	Partial	Failures
Prednisone	1 (1/2)		1 (1/2)
Vincristine + rubidomycin	1 (6^+)		
Vincristine + prednisone	1 (6)		1 (1)
6-mercaptopurine + prednisone		1 (1)	
Methotrexate + prednisone			1 (1)
Methotrexate + folinic acid	2 (1, 10)		1 (1/2)
Rubidomycin + prednisone	1 (5)		
Vincristine + rubidomycin + prednisone	4 (8^+, 7, 1, 1)	2 (3, 1)	3 (1/2, 1/2, 1)
Cyclophosphamide + vincristine + prednisone	1 (8)		
L-asparaginase + vincristine + prednisone	2 (1/2, 1/2)		
Vinblastine + methyl-hydrazine + T.E.M. + prednisone		1 (4)	
L-asparaginase + vincristine + rubidomycin + prednisone	1 (3^+)		
Total	14 / 25	4 / 25	7 / 25

Summary

Blastic crisis is the possible end evolution of some cases of malignant hematopoietic diseases: i. e., lymphoblastosarcomas, reticulosarcomas, chronic myelocytic leukemia, polycytemia vera.

Blastic crisis in the two kinds of malignant lymphomas (i. e. histioblastosarcomas and lymphoblastosarcomas) is relatively frequent: leukemic syndrome is about 3 times more frequent after lymphoblastosarcoma than after histioblastosarcoma. Its prognosis is very bad after histioblastosarcoma, but rather better after lymphoblastosarcoma.

New drug combinations must be tried to improve the prognosis.

References

Mathé, G., Gerard-Marchant, R., Texier, J. L., Schlumberger, J. R., Berumen, L., Paintrand, M.: Les deux variétés de «réticulosarcomes» du tissu lymphoïde, histiocytaire et histioblastique. En préparation.

— Tubiana, M., Calman, F., Schlumberger, J. R., Berumen, L., Choquet, C., Cattan, A., Schneider, M.: Les syndromes de leucémie aigue (SLA) apparaissant au cours de l'évolution des hématosarcomes et des leucémies chroniques (analyse clinique). Nouv. Rev. franç. Hémat. 7, 543 (1967).

IV. Conclusion

Long-Term Survivors in Acute Leukemia[1]

J. H. BURCHENAL

Division of Applied Therapy, Sloan-Kettering Institute for Cancer Research
and the Department of Medicine, Memorial Hospital for Cancer and Allied Diseases
New York, N. Y.

It is obvious from the many publications on the subject that long-term survivors, defined as those patients who survive either with or without evidence of the disease for more than 5 years from the diagnosis, do occur in acute leukemia [1—5]. Previous studies have shown that those patients surviving for 5 years have a 50% chance of surviving indefinitely [6]. Most of those who relapse will do so between the 5th and 8th years, and only a very few after the 9th year. For instance, of the 101 patients reported as 5-year survivors in 1964, 64 were living and well at that time with no evidence of the disease. In the ensuing 4 years, 6 of these had relapsed so that there were 58 out of 101 surviving with no evidence of the disease, or an annual drop-off of approximately 2.5% [7].

The early studies of the Long-Term Survivors Registry of the Acute Leukemia Task Force showed only the number of long-term survivors that was reported, but not the number of cases from which they were derived. Thus our fraction showing the incidence of long-term remissions is lacking a denominator. More recent studies, however, have begun to supply this missing factor. ZUELZER's [8] series of 229 consecutive children with acute lymphoblastic leukemia treated by the cyclic form of chemotherapy is the basic study against which all series showing increased long-term survivors must be judged. As can be seen from Table 1, he had 38% survivors at 2 years, 20% at 3 years, 8% at 4 years, and 4.3% at 5 years. A small series which shows some improvement is that of SELAWRY [9, 10], where of 21 patients treated with large-dose intermittent intramuscular methotrexate, 14% were alive and well at 4 years and also at 5 years. HENDERSON [11] has reported that intensive therapy with the VAMP [12] and BIKE program has increased the survivors to 25% at 4 years, and that similar but longer continued intensive therapy in the POMP [13] program has increased the percentage of survivors to 38% at 3 years. Life table analysis estimates of the 4-year survivors of this series, however, are between 15 and

[1] These studies were supported in part by National Cancer Institute Grants CA-08748 and CA-05826 and American Cancer Society Grant T-45.

Table 1. *Acute lymphoblastic leukemia*

Series	Total patients	Percentage of patients who have survived			
		2 years	3 years	4 years	5 years
Cyclic (ZUELZER)	229	38	20	8	4.3
VAMP & BIKE (FREIREICH et al.)	27	50		25 [a]	
POMP (HENDERSON)	35		38 [a]		
Intermittent MTX (SELAWRY)	21			14	14
Leukemia group B 1964—1965	247	42 [b]	25 [b]	14 [b]	
Leukemia group B 1966—1967	309	51 [b]	32 [b]		
Leukemia group B Protocol 6601-D	53	73 [b]			

[a] Approximate figures.
[b] Life table projection.

25%, thus perhaps no better than the less long continued VAMP and BIKE programs.

Two particularly interesting series are those of Acute Leukemia Group B, as reported by HOLLAND [14]. In this group of patients treated from 1964 and 1965, there were 247 with 42% survivors at 2 years and 25% at 3 years by life-table projection. Of the 309 patients treated between 1966 and 1967, there were 51% 2-year survivors. The more recent figures given here by HOLLAND [14] show that this wave of survivors is now 32% at the 3-year period and is continuing to remain appreciably higher than the Zuelzer figures. Of particular interest is a series of 53 patients in the 66—67 group (6601-D) who were treated with one specific form of chemotherapy: vincristine and prednisone induction, intensive short-course methotrexate consolidation interspersed with periodic inducer doses of prednisone and vincristine. Of this group, the life-table survival estimate at 2 years is 73% [14]. It is important to state that in none of these series except ZUELZER's and SELAWRY's have all patients completed the 5-year observation period. Thus in each series there are still patients alive who may yet survive to the 5-year mark, and, although it is too early to compare the 5-year survivals, it appears likely that with newer and more intensive forms of therapy a significantly higher percentage of 5-year survivors will be achieved.

If we then add to this the effects of L-asparaginase (A-ase) in producing temporary remissions in many patients resistant to all conventional therapy and the occasional long-term unmaintained remissions obtained with this drug alone or in combination with vincristine, Daunomycin, or cytosine arabinoside and thioguanine [15], there should be an even increased number of 5-year survivors.

In addition to the various new and intensive forms of chemotherapy that have been given, one must consider that these long-term survivors may be due not only to exquisite sensitivity of the leukemic cells to chemotherapy but also perhaps to increased host resistance. The studies of Mathé et al. [16] are of great interest in this regard. They have demonstrated that in a series of 30 patients who were in complete remission following a prolonged course of intensive therapy, non-specific immunization with BCG was followed by a much longer period of disease-free, unmaintained remission. Of the series of 10 controls given no maintenance therapy and no immunotherapy, all had relapsed within 130 days of discontinuing chemotherapy. Of the 20 patients given no maintenance chemotherapy but given immunotherapy with either BCG or injections of allogeneic irradiated leukemic cells, or both, 8 out of 20 were in complete remission 295 to 1150 days following the discontinuance of maintenance chemotherapy. These data strongly suggest a real therapeutic gain by the addition of immunotherapy to chemotherapy.

Thus, with the newer schedules of intensive chemotherapy with conventional agents, the combinations with A-ase, and the addition of immunotherapy, it seems likely that the percentage of 5-year survivors and perhaps of permanent remissions in acute leukemia will be markedly increased.

Summary

Long-term survivors, defined as those patients who are surviving, usually without evidence of disease, for more than 5 years from the diagnosis, do occur in acute leukemia. Previous studies have shown that those patients surviving for five years have a 50% chance of surviving indefinitely. With the newer schedules of intensive chemotherapy with conventional agents, the combinations with asparaginase, and the addition of immunotherapy, it seems likely the percentage of five year survivors and perhaps of permanent remissions in acute leukemia will be markedly increased.

References

1. Burchenal, J. H., Murphy, M. L.: Long-term survivors in acute leukemia. Cancer Res. **25**, 1491—1494 (1965).
2. Dameshek, W., Mitus, W. J.: Seven-year remission in an adult with acute leukemia. New Engl. J. Med. **268**, 870—873 (1963).
3. Brubaker, C. A., Wheeler, H. E., Sonley, M. J., Williams, K. O., Hammond, D.: Cyclic chemotherapy for acute leukemia in children. Blood **21**, 820—821 (1963).
4. Zuelzer, W. W.: Formal discussion: Long-term survivors. Cancer Res. **25**, 1495—1498 (1965).
5. — Implications of long-term survival in acute stem cell leukemia of childhood treated with composite cyclic therapy. Blood **24**, 477—494 (1964).
6. Burchenal, J. H.: Long-term survival in Burkitt's tumor and in acute leukemia. Cancer Res. **27**, 2616—2618 (1967).
7. — Analysis of long-term survival in acute leukemia and Burkitt's tumor—effects to be expected from intensive therapy and asparaginase. Proceedings of the Sixth National Cancer Conference, Denver 1968. Philadelphia: J. B. Lippincott Co. 1970.
8. Zuelzer, W. W.: Therapy of acute leukemia in childhood. In: Proceedings of the International Conference on Leukemia-Lymphoma. Ed.: C. J. D. Zarafonetis. Philadelphia: Lea & Febiger 1968, p. 451.
9. Acute Leukemia Group B: New treatment schedule with improved survival in childhood leukemia. Intermittent parental vs. daily oral administration of methotrexate for maintenance of induced remission. J. Amer. med. Ass. **194**, 75—81 (1965).

10. SELAWRY, O.: Personal communication.
11. HENDERSON, E. S.: Evidence that drugs in multiple combinations have materially advanced the treatment of human malignancies. Cancer Res. Dec. 1969.
12. FREIREICH, E. J., KARON, M., FREI, E. III.: Quadruple combination therapy (VAMP) for acute lymphocytic leukemia of childhood. Proc. Amer. Ass. Cancer Res. **5**, 20 (1964).
13. HENDERSON, E. S., FREIREICH, E. J., KARON, M., ROSSEE, W.: High dose combination chemotherapy in acute lymphocytic leukemia of childhood. Proc. Amer. Ass. Cancer Res. **7**, 30 (1966).
14. HOLLAND, J. F.: Complementary chemotherapy in acute leukemia. This volume, p. 95—108.
15. BURCHENAL, J. H.: Clinical evaluation and future prospects of asparaginase. This volume, p. 20—27.
16. MATHÉ, G., AMIEL, J. L., SCHWARZENBERG, L., SCHNEIDER, M., CATTAN, A., SCHLUMBERGER, J. R., HAYAT, M., DE VASSAL, F.: Active immunotherapy for acute lymphoblastic leukemia. Lancet 1969 **I**, 697—699.

Who Should Treat Acute Leukemia?[1]

J. F. Holland

Operations Office, Suite 2F, 651 Elm Street, Buffalo, New York 14203

With 2 Figures

Acute leukemia is a generic term representing a variety of closely related diseases characterized by abnormal proportions of immature hematopoietic cells, often of abnormal morphology. These diseases in their untreated state eventually prove fatal, nearly always within one year.

Their etiologies or etiology are unknown, and form the basis for a vast spectrum of fundamental research.

The treatment of acute leukemia can be divided into three rough historical stages: 1) before 1947, the era of despair with no effective treatment, 2) from 1947 to 1963, the advent of chemotherapy, and with the failure to find a curative drug, the era of palliation, and 3) since 1963, when induction therapies, complementary treatments, including consolidation, intensification, maintenance and inducer dosing, the multiple combinations of drugs, the appearance of new chemotherapeutic agents, and the beginnings of successful immunotherapy have made palliation alone too mean a goal. Chemotherapeutic cure is now a realistic target. Burchenal has gathered over a hundred individuals from the world's experience, many of whom, now in excess of 10 years without evident disease, would be considered cured [1]. Thus, we are not considering an ethereal proposition, but the implementation of a realistic possibility.

To mount a strategy for chemotherapeutic cure of acute leukemia requires enormous resources. Supplies of proven drugs are necessary as well as new drugs at the earliest stages of their potential contribution. Supply of skilled personnel is critical, not only senior individuals whose knowledge and experience blend into wisdom, but young vigorous investigators with good ideas, sometimes new, often iconoclastic, who have the tenacity, energy and time to pursue their implementation on a day to day basis. Striving toward a chemotherapeutic cure requires exceptional support of the patient during predictable crises of the disease. A resourceful blood bank with capacity to provide blood components for therapy is imperative. Erythrocyte and thrombocyte replacement are essential and successful means of support. Granulocyte and lymphocyte transfusions may soon prove as practicable and

[1] The investigations on which this paper is based were conducted by members of the Acute Leukemia Group B and supported by Public Health Service Research Grants No. CA 2599, CA 10456, CA 7918, CA 3927, CA 4737, CA 4326, CA 5462, CA 11028, CA 4646, CA 3735, CA 4457, CA 7968, CA 8025, CA 5923, CA 7757, CA 8080 from the National Cancer Institute.

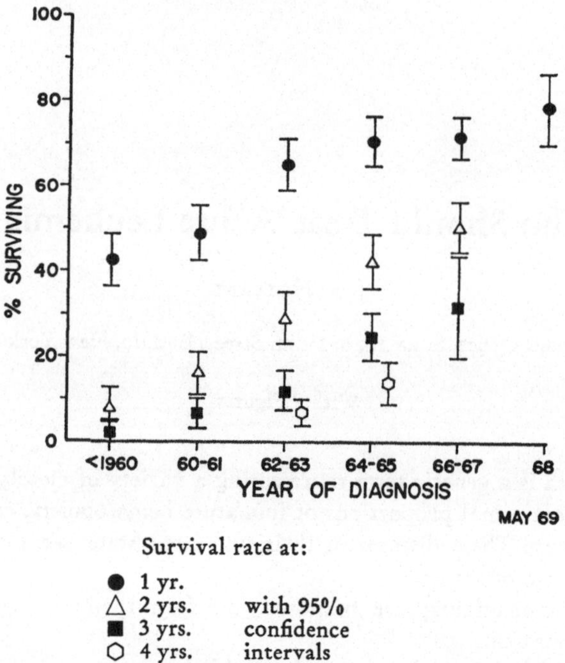

Fig. 1. Survival rates with 95% confidence intervals in all patients with acute lymphocytic leukemia under age 20 treated on study programs by the investigators of Acute Leukemia Group B. The increase in the per cent surviving 1, 2, 3 and 4 years appears to be rising in a nearly parallel ascent. The principal drugs during these studies were methotrexate, 6-mercaptopurine, vincristine, and prednisone. Study protocols were changed several times during the decade, always trying to use the best of what had just been learned.

as necessary. Human leukocytic antigenic typing will be as important in assuring compatibility and effective function of these blood components as was grouping for erythrocytes.

Infection in acute leukemia is commonplace and is that single group of diseases which most often determines mortality. A highly efficient bacteriology laboratory characterizes all centers where progress in chemotherapy of leukemia as occurred. Partial and progressive control of bacteriological infection has placed increasing stress on effective recognition and therapy of fungal, viral, mycoplasma and protozoal infections. All these microorganisms may have clinical importance in patients with acute leukemia and prevent the attainment of control, when they interpose lethal challenge which is unsuccessfully met.

If the requisites for a vigorous attack on acute leukemia, at a minimum, are defined as drugs, personnel, blood bank and microbiological resources, one could question what is lacking for immediate success in attaining cure. It might be argued that the proper concepts and tools are not yet at hand and that a remarkable highly specific drug eventually will appear. This contravenes the fact, however, that some chemotherapeutic cures have probably already been obtained. Recent research data demonstrate that there is still much more therapeutic advantage to be gained from the therapies at hand when properly used, Fig. 1. Such innovations are not likely to occur in the usual hospital or physician's office.

Rather, the proper setting for attempting chemotherapeutic cure requires a critical mass of intellect and of service personnel. Many of the world's great universities and cancer research centers have even found their own resources too limited to sustain as highly productive an activity alone as they can in concert. The design of chemotherapeutic studies and their execution requires a major time commitment of many individuals of high competence.

If one were to accept the inevitability of the fatality of acute leukemia, there would be little reason to leave the comforts of one's family physician and the emotional supports and reassurance of one's community hospital. There is a different kind of emotional support which comes from the specialized treatment center, however, if one accepts the proposition that acute leukemia can be cured and some day will reproducibly be curable in the majority. Some children presently under treatment have, as a group, such extended survival that there will in all probability be cured individuals among them. Chemotherapeutic results in adults have lagged somewhat behind the children, but the availability of several active drugs in leukemia centers, compared to the small selection in practice nonetheless provides optimal opportunity for remission at the centers.

The best organizational framework for success appears to me to be a cooperative venture between the patient's own physician and his closest investigational center in leukemia therapy. In a major city, such a center might be only 100 blocks away and nonetheless, because of the patterns of medical practice, as remote as if it were across an ocean. At the outset of acute leukemia, while the disease is florid, and when the most critical chemotherapy and supportive care is required, I believe the patient should be admitted to the closest center well-equipped to meet these requirements. Part of the task is to formulate a program of care which is consonant with the best in research which has already been accomplished, and which seeks to find even better approaches. The definition of the center is of course, circumstantially dependent. In a metropolis it would likely be in a large university hospital or research institution that one would find the critical mass of personnel and resources. One would expect the practicing hematologist, internist, or pediatrician to arrange for the hospitalization of his patients there, and upon discharge after initial intensive treatment, to coordinate his activities with the programs of the center. The center may be obliged to provide education, drugs and consultations with the physician in order to aid him in his mission.

In a remote smaller city, the center might indeed constitute the same type of physician and small hospital from which patients would be transferred in the metropolis. Obviously, not every patient from the rural areas can or will travel to the university or research center for treatment, irrespective of the probable advantages. In such circumstances, the practicing hematologist has a substantial responsibility to keep himself current with the best of published information, with drugs that are available to him and to achieve the maximum support from blood bank and microbiological labtoratories to aid him.

If, however, the leukemia center cares for the hospitalization portions of a patient's illness and shares the management during ambulatory phases with a patient's physician, considerable benefits should accrue to all concerned. The supply of patients would be ample to conduct investigation to seek improvements above our present levels of achievement. It also would allow access to the patient in his first treatment

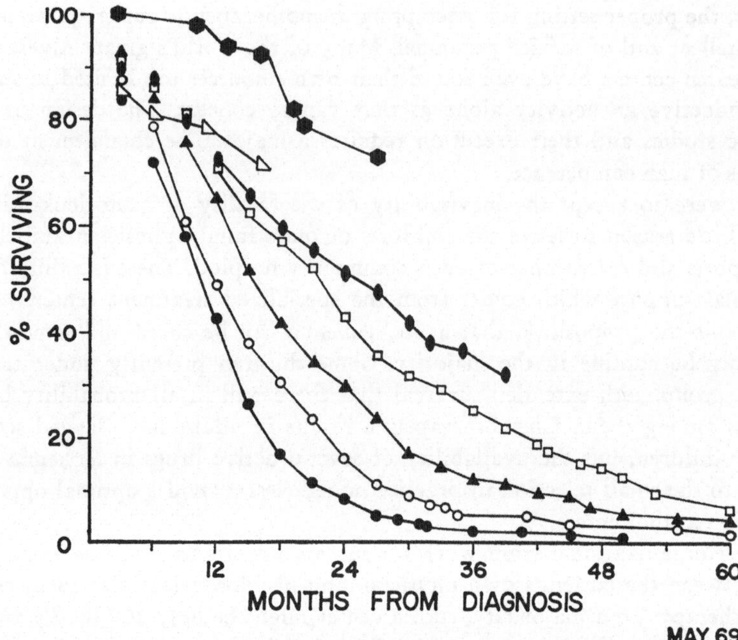

Fig. 2. Survival experience plotted by the life table method in 1390 patients with acute lymphocytic leukemia under age 20 treated by the investigators of Acute Leukemia Group B. Before 1960 no child survived 5 years. Successive experience and projections for recent years indicate that increasing numbers will reach this point in time, an obvious prerequisite for identifying the child in whom the disease may be eradicated. Regimen D, a program using vincristine, prednisone, and methotrexate in intensive courses as the first treatment, is a component portion of the 309 children in 66—67.

	Diagnosis	Patients
●	ā 60	255
○	60—61	227
▲	62—63	234
□	64—65	247
⬮	66—67	309
▷	68	118
⬢	Regimen D	53

which appears of such critical importance. The patient would benefit from the participation of a leukemia center in his care by a factor as great as the capacities of the center exceed those of the single practicing physician. Lastly, the referring physician would also benefit by virtue of his own participation in the research, and the presumptive advantages to his patient, who, if improperly managed, will succumb all the sooner. Leukemia, after all, is not bread-and-butter practice but a challenge of great magnitude that society as a whole has repeatedly identified as a scourge.

Data which demonstrate higher frequency and greater duration of remissions, lengthening survival and a possibility of some cured patients among the survivors have been presented in recent years (Fig. 2). Since leukemia can be cured in special experimental circumstances, and cure is possible in man, we must not slacken the pace. Indeed, the progress in acute leukemia serves as a model system for other cancer therapy in man. Principles derived from leukemia have successfully found their way into the chemotherapy of other human cancer.

Today's patients and today's society have a vital interest in specialized centers of research at both clinical and fundamental levels. One can hope for the day when such investigations will lead to prevention of acute leukemia. Preventive measures then could be given routinely to infants in the physician's office or a public health clinic. It hardly seems likely, however, that once the disease is developed, its treatment will ever be simple or without the need for coordinated approach between experts at the highest level of specialization, laboratories with vast resources, and the patient's family physician.

Summary

Leukemia treatment is founded on the possibility that eradication of the disease is a realistic objective.

Increasing intensity of treatment with innovation in treatment techniques has led to longer survival. The requirements for such aggressive treatment are drugs, a critical mass of specialized professional personnel, a blood bank with capacity to provide cell components, and microbiological resources. These several factors constitute a leukemia center. Such a center is best able to manage the patient during crises of leukemia, sharing responsibility with the patient's physician during ambulatory periods.

References

1. Burchenal, J. H.: Long term survivors in acute leukemia and Burkitt's tumor. Cancer 21, 595—599 (1968).
2. — This symposium.

Treatment of Acute Leukemia

G. Mathé

Institut de Cancérologie et d'Immunogénétique, Hôpital Paul-Brousse 14, avenue Paul-Vaillant Couturier, 94-Villejuif, France

The communications presented at this conference have confirmed that progress is continuing in the treatment of acute leukaemia.

This progress has been, firstly, in the introduction of new methods of therapy: the importance of asparaginase has been confirmed; the effectiveness of ICRF 159 (dioxopiperazine propane) is rare but demonstrated; though poly IC has not been used yet in clinical trials to assess its action in man, it does provide an interferon inducer for therapeutic research. Dr. Henderson gave a very hopeful list. Adoptive immunotherapy from bone marrow grafts or lymphocyte transfusions can be added to chemotherapy; but, most important, is active immunotherapy, either specific or non-specific; at least two adjuvants appear to be able to be available to day for man.

The second direction of our progress is in what I like to call "operational research", which is the study of how to obtain the maximum benefit from drugs and other methods of therapy. Knowledge of the cell kinetics of leukaemic cells, haematopoietic stem cells, and immunologically competent cells would seem to be able to help in finding the best method to give therapy.

It goes without saying, that the kinetics should be studied not only in animals but in man. And well conducted, comparative therapeutic trials, based on sound scientific principles, are of paramount importance. To achieve this aim, collaboration between of hospitals, both within a country and internationally, are necessary. The meeting to day of a co-operative group of the E.O.R.T.C. and American representatives, can be thought of as the beginning of transatlantic co-operation, the forerunner of world-wide collaboration.

It is not sufficient just to work out the conditions to achieve the maximum efficiency for each individual drugs: strategic research is concerned with finding the best form of therapy, using all the drugs that are available, and determining the best strategy of using them in combination.

Chemotherapy obeys the law of the first kinetics order, that is a given dose can only destroy a given percentage of leukaemic cells; it cannot destroy them all. On the other hand, active immunotherapy seems to be able to eradicate completely a population of tumour cells, but only when the number of tumour cells in this population is very small, and has no action when the number of tumour cells is high. This has suggested to us that the following strategy should be employed: chemotherapy to induce a remission, followed by complementary chemotherapy to reduce the persisting tumour cell number, then active immunotherapy. Other schemes are studied by Dr. HOLLAND, more numerous than his personal collection of wonderful ties.

For operational and strategic research to be profitable for each patient, to enable him to have the best chance afforded by using the most effective therapy in the most efficient manner, requires considerable organisation. There must be adequate ancilliary services (pathogen-free rooms, leucocyte and platelet given intensive therapy), and the clinics should deal with large numbers of leukaemic patients.

It is highly desirable, from scientific and ethical standpoints, that patients suffering from acute leukaemia should be treated in special cancer services, as has been suggested by Dr. HOLLAND, and they should be referred there at the onset of the illness.

Do we have in our hands to-day the methods to cure acute lymphoblastic leukaemia? Certainly not the methods to cure all the patients; may be the methods to cure some; hence, each patient must be given the greatest chance to survive. It is inadmissible that they should not be treated by the most experienced physicians from the time the illness is first discovered.

The time is coming to set up a world-wide organisation for the treatment of acute leukaemia. The demand for personal publications can, perhaps, be taken to be justification for the basic research workers, but co-operation should aim to give the patients the maximum chance of cure and to forward research applied to the treatment of leukaemia.

To reach this goal, many ways will have to be tried, which will require large sums of money, then more and more money. I must acknowledge the immense effort of the American people in this respect; each inhabitant gives four times more towards cancer research than each Frenchman gives for the whole of medical research. I hope the people of all countries will follow the example of the Americans.

It will not be by chance if, in 1969, we hear that the first men have been on the moon, and we are asking ourselves if some patients with acute lymphoblastic leukaemia and specially the ones Dr. BURCHENAL has spoken above are not cured. Applied research can progress when men and money are committed to the project. It is in biological research that the European countries have the greatest chance of participating effectively, and success in this research would be a source of pride and a true honour for men of our generation, in every country and in every continent.

Monographs already Published

1 SCHINDLER, R., Lausanne: Die tierische Zelle in Zellkultur. DM 16,—; US $ 4.40

2 Neuroblastomas — Biochemical Studies. Edited by C. BOHUON, Villejuif (Symposium). DM 16,—; US $ 4.40

3 HUEPER, W. C., Bethesda: Occupational and Environmental Cancers of the Respiratory System. DM 34,—; US $ 9.40

4 GOLDMAN, L., Cincinnati: Laser Cancer Research. DM 16,—; US $ 5.00

5 METCALF, D., Melbourne: The Thymus. Its Role in Immune Responses, Leukaemia Development and Carcinogenesis. DM 24,—; US $ 6.60

6 Malignant Transformation by Viruses. Edited by W. H. KIRSTEN, Chicago (Symposium). DM 32,—; US $ 8.80

7 MOERTEL, CH. G., Rochester: Multiple Primary Malignant Neoplasms. Their Incidence and Significance. DM 18,—; US $ 5.00

8 New Trends in the Treatment of Cancer. Edited by L. MANUILA, S. MOLES, and P. RENTCHNICK, Geneva. DM 32,—; US $ 8.80

9 LINDENMANN, J., Zürich, and P. A. KLEIN, Gainesville/Florida: Immunological Aspects of Viral Oncolysis. DM 18,—; US $ 5.00

10 NELSON, R. S., Houston: Radioactive Phosphorus in the Diagnosis of Gastrointestinal Cancer. DM 15,—; US $ 4.20

11 FREEMAN, R. G., and J. M. KNOX, Houston: Treatment of Skin Cancer. DM 15,—; US $ 4.50

12 LYNCH, H. T., Houston: Hereditary Factors in Carcinoma. DM 24,—; US $ 6.60

13 Tumours in Children. Edited by H. B. MARSDEN, and J. K. STEWARD, Manchester. DM 72,—; US $ 18.00

14 ODARTCHENKO, N., Lausanne: Production cellulaire érythropoïétique. DM 28,—; US $ 7.70

15 SOKOLOFF, B., Lakeland/Florida: Carcinoid and Serotonin. DM 24,—; US $ 6.60

16 JACOBS, M. L., Duarte/California: Malignant Lymphomas and their Management. DM 18,—; US $ 5.10

17 Normal and Malignant Cell Growth. Edited by R. J. M. FRY, Argonne, M. L. GRIEM, Argonne, and W. H. KIRSTEN, Chicago (Symposium). DM 56,80; US $ 14.20

18 ANGLESIO, E., Torino: The Treatment of Hodgkin's Disease. DM 24,—; US $ 6.60

19 BANNASCH, P., Würzburg: The Cytoplasm of Hepatocytes during Carcinogenesis. DM 32,—; US $ 8.80

20 Rubidomycin. A new Agent against Leukemia. Edited by J. BERNARD, R. PAUL, M. BOIRON, C. JACQUILLAT, and R. MARAL, Paris. DM 48,—; US $ 13.20

21 Scientific Basis of Cancer Chemotherapy. Edited by G. MATHÉ, Villejuif (Symposium). DM 28,—; US $ 7.70

22 KOLDOVSKÝ, P., Philadelphia: Tumor Specific Transplantation Antigen. DM 24,—; US $ 6.60

23 FUCHS, W. A., Bern, J. W. DAVIDSON, Toronto, and H. W. FISCHER, Ann Arbor: Lymphography in Cancer. DM 76,—; US $ 21.00

24 HAYWARD, J. L., London: Hormonal Research in Human Breast Cancer. DM 34,—; US $ 9.40

25 ROY-BURMAN, P., Los Angeles: Analogues of Nucleic Acid Components. Mechanisms of Action. DM 28,—; US $ 7.70

26 Tumors of the Liver. Edited by G. T. PACK and A. H. ISLAMI, New York. DM 56,—; US $ 15.40

27 SZYMENDERA, J., Warsaw: Bone Mineral Metabolism in Cancer. DM 32,—; US $ 8.80

28 MEEK, E. S., Bristol: Antitumour and Antiviral Substances of Natural Origin. DM 16,—; US $ 4.40

29 Aseptic Environments and Cancer Treatment. Edited by G. MATHÉ, Villejuif (Symposium). DM 22,—; US $ 6.10

30 Advances in the Treatment of Acute (Blastic) Leukemias. Edited by G. MATHÉ, Villejuif (Symposium). DM 38,—; US $ 10.50

In Production

31 DENOIX, P., Villejuif: Treatment of Malignant Breast Tumors: Indications and Results. DM 48,—; US $ 13.20

32 NELSON, R. S., Houston: Endoscopy in Gastric Cancer. DM 48,—; US $ 13.20

33 Experimental and Clinical Effects of L-Asparaginase. Edited by E. GRUNDMANN, Wuppertal-Elberfeld, and H. F. OETTGEN, New York (Symposium). DM 58,—; US $ 16.—

34 ENDO, H., Fukuoka, T. ONO, Tokyo, T. SUGIMURA, Tokyo: Chemistry and Biological Actions of 4-Nitroquinoline 1-oxide

In Preparation

ACKERMANN, N. B., Boston: Use of Radioisotopic Agents in the Diagnosis of Cancer

BOIRON, M., Paris: The Viruses of the Leukemia-sarcoma Complex

CAVALIERE, R., A. ROSSI-FANELLI, B. MONDOVI, and G. MORICCA, Roma: Selective Heat Sensitivity of Cancer Cells

CHIAPPA, S., Milano: Endolymphatic Radiotherapy in Malignant Lymphomas

Cutane paraneoplastische Syndrome. Edited by J. J. HERZBERG, Bremen (Symposium)

GRUNDMANN, E., Wuppertal-Elberfeld: Morphologie und Cytochemie der Carcinogenese

IRLIN, I. S., Moskva: Mechanisms of Viral Carcinogenesis

LANGLEY, F. A., and A. C. CROMPTON, Manchester: Epithelial Abnormalities of the Cervix Uteri

MATHÉ, G., Villejuif: L'Immunothérapie des Cancers

NEWMAN, M. K., Detroit: Neuropathies and Myopathies Associated with Occult Malignancies

OGAWA, K., Osaka: Ultrastructural Enzyme Cytochemistry of Azo-dye Carcinogenesis

PENN, I., Denver: Malignant Lymphomas in Transplant Patients

WEIL, R., Lausanne: Biological and Structural Properties of Polyoma Virus and its DNA

WILLIAMS, D. C., Caterham, Surrey: The Basis for Therapy of Hormon Sensitive Tumours

WILLIAMS, D. C., Caterham, Surrey: The Biochemistry of Metastasis